Life, Cancer and God

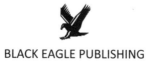

BLACK EAGLE PUBLISHING

"And you shall know the truth,
and the truth shall make you free."

— John 8:32

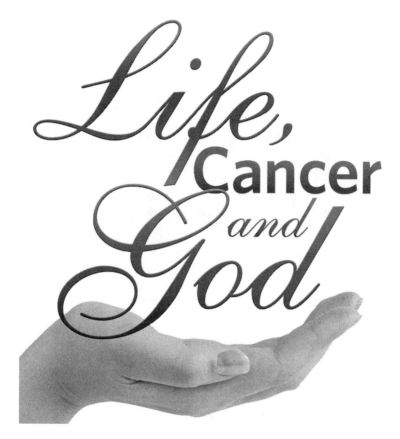

Life, Cancer and God

Healing Your
Body, Soul & Spirit

Paula Black *and* Capt. Dale Black, PhD

BLACK EAGLE PUBLISHING

Cover design by George Foster Book Cover Design
Editing and page design by ChristianEditingServices.com

Published by Black Eagle Publishing, Inc.
140 E. Stetson Ave., #222
Hemet, CA 92543

Printed in the United States of America

Library of Congress Cataloging-in-Publication Data is available upon request.

ISBN 978-0-09885346-0-5 (softcover)
ISBN 978-0-09885346-3-6 (hardcover)

10 9 8 7 6 5 4 3 2 1

BLACK EAGLE PUBLISHING

A special thank you to

Lorraine Day, M.D.

By personally sharing her vast medical background and hands-on knowledge about how to reverse cancer, Dr. Lorraine Day was instrumental in saving my life. Her courage to stand up to the pressures of conventional medical protocol—at great personal cost—in an effort to find and share the truth about cancer is both commendable and praiseworthy. She has given life and health to thousands and is one of the most outstanding women I have ever met.

**This book is lovingly dedicated
to three fabulous women in my life:**

To my mother and friend, Juanita Hubbard, who
was a shining example in the face of her own battle
with cancer. She walked in victory . . .
I walked in her footsteps.

To my daughter, Kara Black, the joy and light of my life.
She is my inspiration to hold the bar high.

To my sister, Marna Whitley, a loving friend and confidante.
Her unconditional love and support are available
whenever I need them.

Authors' and Publisher's Disclaimer

The information contained in this book originates from personal discovery by the authors and is an expression of their personal journey. Dale Black and Paula Black are ministers and businesspeople, not physicians. The authors are merely presenting their findings, as would an investigative journalist. A conscientious effort has been made to present only information that is accurate and truthful. However, the authors cannot be held responsible for inaccuracies that may be found in their source material nor do they assume responsibility for how this material is used.

It is your right to consult with a healthcare professional. It is also your God-given and legal right to treat yourself, but you must assume all responsibility. None of the information in this book should be construed as "medical advice," and in no way should anyone infer that the authors are practicing medicine.

Anyone who has—or suspects they have—cancer or any other chronic disease, should consult with a healthcare professional. Also, before starting any new vitamins, supplements, diet, or exercise program, a healthcare professional should be consulted.

The alternative non-toxic approach depicted in this book has not been evaluated by the United States Food and Drug Administration (FDA). Any information contained herein is not intended to diagnose, treat, cure, or prevent disease. The publisher and authors disclaim liability for any medical outcomes that may occur as a result of applying the methods described in this book.

Contents

FREE GIFT - Paula's "Jump Start Plan"
Jump start your health with your FREE GIFT (valued at $30).
Receive one Healthy Juice Recipe, one Faith-Building Bible Promise,
and one "Heart-Talk" Affirmation from Paula
by email EVERY DAY for 30 days.

Send email to: jumpstart@lifecancerandgod.com

Introduction
by Paula Black

⟿

In the prime of my life—as a wife, mother, businesswoman, and co-pastor of a church—I heard the dreaded words: "It's cancer". Doctors gave me just three to six months to live. With my husband Dale's help, I began researching everything I could about my fatal disease. We met with doctors and oncologists. We talked with cancer patients and their families. We tirelessly researched every conventional and alternative cancer treatment available. But mostly, we prayed.

Eventually, I would find a combination of methods that treated the root causes of my disease, not just the symptoms. Against my doctor's advice, I followed my own newly discovered path, which I call the Body-Soul-Spirit approach. I learned how to strengthen my body's immune system while simultaneously deepening my faith in God. By blending SPIRITUAL truths with NATURAL remedies, I got well. What I learned and acted on saved my life.

In the twenty-four months it has taken to write this book, 1,144,800 people have died of cancer in the United States alone. The American Cancer Society tells us that one in two men and one in three women will get cancer in their lifetime. They also report that 4,500 Americans are diagnosed with cancer and 1,590 die of cancer *every day*. Cancer is an epidemic that touches all of us.

Even though the above numbers are getting worse, not better, cancer no longer scares me—nor do I fear its return. You will understand why by the time you have finished reading this book.

My journey was frightening, exhilarating, and challenging. I had to make life-and-death choices, to consider the consequences my husband and children faced, and to contemplate the real possibility of death by cancer. During this process, my husband and I became experts on cancer. Often I went cross-grain to the medical establishment, which was unsettling and scary but ultimately proved to be the right choice for me.

Many have called me a cancer *survivor*. I reject that label. I didn't simply survive cancer—I am *cured* of cancer.

When I was diagnosed, Dale was my rock, offering me unconditional love and support. He became my head cheerleader and my counselor. His previous experience as the only survivor of an airplane crash gave him an astounding ability to see life through a spiritual lens, along with the history of overcoming life-threatening injuries. I do not believe I would be alive today if it were not for his help in my fight against cancer.

Dale also became my full-time cancer researcher. As a career airline pilot instructor, he spent decades researching and teaching complex aeronautical science and jet aircraft systems to pilots and engineers. When I was diagnosed with cancer, Dale put these well-honed skills to valuable use, digging tirelessly for the information I would need to reverse my disease.

The decision to share my story has been both challenging and rewarding. So why do I feel compelled to tell of my battle with cancer now? So far, Dale and I have lost over forty family members and very close friends to this horrible disease. Every family seems to be touched in some way by cancer. And most have only heartbreak and loss as a result. I knew that if writing this book could help even one person find his or her own way of escape, I had to be willing.

Throughout this book, I have attempted to be authentic, vulnerable, and open. Like me or not, you will learn who I really am. Dale and I wrote our dialogues and interactions in the same way we act and talk in our real lives. You may not agree with some of our reactions or our decisions, but inside these pages we candidly reveal who we are—the good, the bad, and the ugly. Be prepared for Dale and me to talk about God often. You see, God is an integral part of our daily lives and there is simply no way to exclude Him from my story, nor would I want to.

The book you are about to read is based on my true story. The events are real as well as the characters, but I have taken some liberties to condense the telling for clarity. The names of some people have been changed to protect their privacy. The conversations related within the story have been drawn from our best recollections of those discussions. For ease of understanding, literary license has been used with the character of Dr. Cohen, also known as "the doc." She is a compilation of several real people—two medical doctors and two nutritionists with whom Dale and I met, plus three authors and several healthcare professionals Dale interviewed for the research he did on my behalf.

In an effort to help the reader understand some of the points discussed in this book, a few of the "expert" quotes used to convey certain ideas, or to provide better clarity, are from sources that became available after my event occurred.

You may be reading this book because you enjoy an inspirational story or desire to learn what it's like to battle cancer. Possibly you or a loved one has just been diagnosed with cancer or another chronic disease and are searching for help and hope. Whatever the reason, it's likely this book will give you more than you expect. But brace yourself. What you are about to read you may find shocking. You won't find the information in this book discussed in the mainstream media, nor talked about in your doctor's office.

I hope you'll find my story compelling and educational. I stayed the course with my Body-Soul-Spirit approach, without chemotherapy and without radiation. Eventually, my advanced-stage cancer was gone. I got my life back.

And now . . . told for the first time since this happened seventeen years ago, here is my story.

Chapter 1

The Big Shock

"Open your eyes, Paula. Wake up. Can you hear me?"

Irritating words muscled into the black void of my mind as my eyelids struggled to open against an invisible pressure. Sights and sounds slowly crept in, bringing more questions than answers. *This looks like a hospital, but why am I here? And why is it so cold?*

I tried to pull the blanket closer, but my efforts were sabotaged by a shockwave of pain shooting through my chest.

A familiar voice cut through the fog. "How are you feeling, sweetheart?" I sighed in relief as my husband gently held my hand and kissed my forehead.

"I'm so glad you're here." I squeezed his hand and couldn't let go. "I'm cold . . . and so thirsty. Can you get me a drink?" *Was that really my voice?* It was raspy, so unfamiliar.

"I'll be right back," Dale whispered, gently prying my fingers loose.

The nurse inspected the tubes and gauges, then scribbled notes on my chart. "Paula, are you in any pain?"

I tried to move slightly to shift my body, but pain tore through my chest. "Yes," I managed to gasp. "Yes. Can you give me something? And can I get another blanket please? I'm freezing."

Within moments, a heated blanket was releasing its soothing warmth over me. I could see Dale, wearing a boyish grin, approaching with a plastic cup of water. He bent the straw and gently probed it through my parched lips. I didn't stop drinking until the slurping signaled I had emptied the cup. Water had never tasted better.

With my immediate needs met, I returned my focus to the *whats* and *whys*. I had been through some type of surgery . . . that was obvious. Blazing pain still smoldered in my breast as a reminder. *Oh, yes. I came to the hospital for a lumpectomy. A large mass in my left breast. I remember now. The surgeon was going to remove the tumor. What did they find? Was the tumor benign? It had to be. There's no way I have cancer. Not me.*

If anyone had answers, it would be Dale. After twenty-five years of marriage, I knew him well. He'd dig and pry in his relentless search for the truth. Besides, I could always read his face. My barrage of questions began. "What did they find? Do you know anything yet? Has anyone talked to you?"

Dale hesitated and for a split second his eyes darted away. *Not a good sign.* He locked his gaze on mine and forced a smile. "Everything's going to be fine, Paula. Remember, God wants you well—and He's the final authority."

Comforting words—but a shaky voice. I studied his face. Dale was frightened. My cool, calm, faith-filled husband was afraid. *Right now I wish I didn't know him so well. He's trying to be brave, but he knows something.*

"Dale, tell me everything. What did the doctor say? What do you know?"

"Let's wait a little while, honey. Give your head a chance to clear. You barely know where you are. I'll tell you all the details later, but not now. Just remember: Everything is going to be just fine."

"I know you, Dale. You're stalling." *Are his eyes watering? Is he holding back tears?* Gently touching his arm, I asked again in a softer voice, "Tell me, honey. What did the doctor find?"

I tried to brace myself while Dale appeared to be gathering his strength. It took him several seconds to pull himself together, but the seconds seemed like minutes, and in that time, I knew my life hung in the balance.

Dale covered my hand with his. At last, he uttered, "It's malignant, Paula. It's cancer."

My heart stopped. I died inside. Dale spoke some more, but I didn't hear the words. His mouth was moving, but it was all distant, muffled noise to me. I was blind, deaf, and dumb with shock.

Finally, I managed to focus on what Dale was saying. "The lump was much larger than the doctor originally thought, sweetheart. He couldn't get it all. The tumor has already spread too much. He needs to do additional surgery. As soon as possible. He recommends that your entire breast be removed . . . as well as some of the lymph nodes under your arm."

Is he finished? Please, God, let him be finished. I don't want to hear any more.

Dale could see the anguish in my face. "I'm so sorry, Paula." Tears trickled from his eyes. More silence. He was giving me time to absorb the news. Time I needed.

"Is there any good news?" I said at last.

"Of course, sweetheart, absolutely! The doctor says there's reason to be hopeful. He believes if you have the full-scale chemotherapy and radiation treatments, as well as another surgery, well, then there's a good chance you'll get well. Now, he didn't give us any guarantees, of course, and he cautioned against getting our hopes too high. At the same time, he thinks if you'll let them do the whole nine yards—I mean everything—there's a good possibility they can get rid of the cancer."

My face fell in crushing disappointment. *That's the good news?* "Oh, Dale, I can't believe it. I was so sure the lump would be benign—that I wouldn't actually have cancer." My voice pitched higher and my words trembled. "How could God allow this to happen? I figured we'd do this lumpectomy thing and it would all be over." I turned away and swallowed hard, trying to keep my emotions from exploding.

> **And we know that all things work together for good to those who love God, to those who are the called according to His purpose.**
>
> Romans 8:28

"I know it's overwhelming, honey. I am so sorry. But remember what you and I already know. God wants you well. That's a fact. Remember, His Word tells us that all things work together for good to those who love God and are called according to His purpose. Don't forget that promise, sweetheart. At the same time . . . I didn't think God would allow this, either."

Why did I push so hard for Dale to tell me all this now? Why didn't I let him wait like he suggested? I felt like I'd been broadsided by a speeding freight train.

"Remember this too, Paula. Though Dr. Anderson is an excellent doctor, he's just a man. He's a human being full of frailty, like all of us. He's not the final authority. God and His Word are the final authority. I know you believe that. And let's not forget that 'by His stripes you are healed.'[1] We have a titanic struggle ahead, but if we're going to win it, we need to remember what is true."

Dale was saying all the right words. Words I'd heard him preach as the pastor of the church we were starting. Words

I knew he believed wholeheartedly. Still, something was different about him. Somehow this battle—maybe because it involved me instead of him—was one he had not been prepared for.

"I know, Dale. I know you're right." Yes, I knew. And I believed God's Word. But at that moment my feelings were stronger than what my head knew. *It's cancer.* How could my world have changed so completely by hearing two little words?

A welcome interruption broke the tension as a nurse approached. "Pastor Black, it's time to move your wife to her room. You can go to the waiting area for now and join her in about thirty minutes after we get her settled in."

The nurse and an orderly began unhooking the monitor and moving the IV. I studied Dale's face as he stepped away, slump-shouldered. I wanted to comfort him. I knew how much he depended on me . . . needed me. *If I die, his world will crash into a million pieces.*

I thought back to when our relationship began. We had been college sweethearts. Dale was recovering from an airplane crash a year earlier and dreaming of becoming an airline pilot. I had been selected for the Pasadena Tournament of Roses Court. We fell in love fast and hard and married soon after we met.

We came from vastly contrasting backgrounds so our relationship had struggled from the beginning. Our mutual commitment to God was our strongest bond when so much else tried to pull us apart. Despite our distinct differences, our love was strong, and neither of us could imagine living without the other. Now, facing this crisis, there was no one I would rather have beside me.

Dale's voice broke as my bed was rolled through the doorway. "I'll see you in a few minutes, honey."

I lifted my hand in a weak wave as he disappeared from view. Usually I tried to be the encourager. Not this time.

Alone with my thoughts, I watched fluorescent lights pass overhead. I could hear the clicking and squeaking of wheels and shoes scuffing on linoleum. A new reality was trying to take root, but I was not ready to let it in. How could I? There was still so much I didn't understand.

I'm a fixer. Once I collect all the facts, even if those facts are bad, given enough time, I'll figure out a plan. I always have. But this? *I have cancer? And apparently it's really bad because the doctor couldn't get it all. And now he wants to remove my entire breast? And lymph nodes? What does that mean anyway? How advanced is it? How much has it spread? Where has it spread?*

The short journey to my room provided a much needed distraction, if only for a few minutes. My bed was wheeled into an oversized elevator that took us up to the fourth floor. As we exited, I could see a bustling nurses' station with a middle-aged woman sitting behind the desk on the telephone while another nurse stood at the counter studying someone's chart. No one paid any attention to me. I was just another patient in the constant parade that marched by hour after hour each day.

The wide hall was dotted with carts, metal IV stands, and supply cupboards. We entered a comfortable room where I was moved onto a bed next to a large window. *Oh good. At least for now I'm the only patient in the room.*

Once I was situated in my new environment, everyone left and I was alone for the first time since hearing I had cancer. Except for occasional sounds from the hall, the room was quiet. I gazed out the large picture window. The sky was fittingly overcast. I wished for rain—the sky could shed the tears I was struggling to hold back. I didn't like anyone to see me cry. Not even Dale. I needed to be strong and capable, and I hated feeling vulnerable. But vulnerable was exactly what I was.

This hadn't been my first experience with a formidable obstacle. But this was different—more intimate, more deadly. *This will be a big one. Cancer is already changing everything.*

In the quiet of my room, I began to revisit my life. Had I lived long enough? It had been a full life for my forty-five years, but there was still so much I wanted to do—so much to live for.

I thought back. Three months after Dale and I were married, we headed to the jungles of northern Peru to work as volunteer missionaries with the primitive Aguaruna Indian tribe. Both of us were adventurers at heart. That mission experience changed us, individually and as a couple. A love for people and missions was born, a love that propelled us into a life of ministry.

I thought about the aviation businesses we had started—training jet pilots and offering jet charter flights. We both loved business but our hearts belonged in ministry, so we packed our lives with both. Dale eventually succeeded at reaching his goal of becoming an airline pilot with a major U.S. carrier. But we still had so many plans . . . so many dreams.

And then there was family. How would this news impact our two children, Eric and Kara? I loved them both so much and wanted to be part of their lives for many more years. Even though they were grown, there were so many important moments ahead. Who would they marry? Who would love my grandchildren like I would? And I knew the most important thing I could do would be to pray for them every day. Life is difficult and prayer would be the best gift I could give them.

There was so much purpose in living, and suddenly I knew I never wanted so badly to live. The fear of disappearing from the lives of the ones I loved was overwhelming. My chest tightened with each thought like a chain being ratcheted to the point of breaking. I could barely breathe as I tried to mentally loosen the invisible band restricting my oxygen. *What is happening to me?* I was breathing but getting no air. *This must be how it feels to suffocate.*

Only twenty minutes had passed since learning I had cancer, but already I knew my life would never be the same. For the first time in years, I was afraid. So much was at stake. Tears began rolling from my eyes. I tried to steel myself but couldn't stop them. Someone could show up at any moment and I didn't want to look weak, but the drops became streams running down the sides of my face, disappearing into my hair and soaking into my pillow.

Thoughts formed like spider webs I couldn't escape. Questions surged past in an unstoppable assembly line. *Do I really have cancer? Could it be true? What does it all mean? What will I have to go through? When will this nightmare be over? Will it kill me? How can I die so young?* So many people I'd known had already died of cancer.

What makes me think I'll be any different?

I wondered how my parents would take the news. We were close. I knew how devastated they'd be if something happened to any of their children. And what about my sister? *This will be really hard on her. We've been through so much together. I can't imagine not having her in my life, and I know she feels the same.*

I tried to gain perspective and slow my mind. I wasn't ready to accept any of this yet. As I struggled to hold back the sobs, desperate words escaped my lips: "Not me, God. Please not me. And not now. Not this way! Not cancer."

Little did I know that my frantic prayer would be answered—in ways I could never have imagined. I was embarking on a journey that would change me—in ways I had no idea needed changing.

CHAPTER 2

Promise

Carts clattered down the hallway while the drone of voices from early morning rounds filtered in. Hospitals are not a place for sleeping. "Good morning, Mrs. Black. How are you feeling?" The nurse studied my chart.

"Okay, I guess. What time is it?"

"Six-fifteen." She unceremoniously yanked back the curtains, robbing me of any privacy, and around my arm went the blood pressure device.

I gazed out the window at the gray overcast that stubbornly hung on. *I don't really have cancer. They probably made a big mistake and today this will all be over.*

I clung to hope. Trying to gather more of it, I recalled how Dale dealt with his life-and-death crisis as the passenger and sole survivor of a catastrophic airplane crash. Early in his aviation career, he and two other pilots were flying a load of cargo when, seconds after takeoff, their twin-engine airplane smashed into a huge, seven-story building. With an impact speed of 135 miles an hour, the plane shattered into a thousand pieces. The three pilots then free-fell 75 feet to the ground.

Although the crash was classified as non-survivable, Dale is still very much alive. *Why? Why did he live and the others die?* I thought I knew. While Dale lay in a coma, he experienced a life-altering journey to heaven—and back. He had gone from life, to death, to life again.

Dale's doctor spelled out a dire prognosis: "If Dale does survive, he'll likely have permanent brain damage from the blunt trauma. That's what killed the other pilots. He'll certainly never walk again. He'll not be able to use his left arm or see out of his right eye. His back is broken in several places. He's broken both legs, both knees, and both ankles. Airplane parts had to be surgically removed from all over his body including his head and face. My biggest concern is his head injuries."

On the morning of the fourth day, Dale emerged from the coma—with a transformed heart. Nothing would be the same for him again—ever.

Eventually, working hand in hand with God and against all odds, he learned to walk, run, and even fly again. *Dale is a walking miracle.*[2]

That's the same God I know. And the Bible says He is no respecter of persons—He shows no partiality.[3] *Wouldn't He be willing to do the same thing for me? Wouldn't God answer my prayers like He answered Dale's?*

And what about my mom? She had breast cancer when she was forty-five.

Mom's tumor was malignant and doctors planned on removing her breast and lymph nodes. While she waited for surgery, she focused on God and studied her Bible. Every time we spoke, she told me God was in the process of healing her. I never saw Mom more zealous for God and His ways than when diagnosed with cancer. I watched her share her faith with complete strangers.

The day of Mom's operation arrived. I had flown up and was with Dad at the hospital. Early that morning we entered Mom's room to see her one last time before surgery. There she was, minutes before her operation, grinning, with a glow of joy about her. *It must be the drugs.*

"The lump is gone! The doctor said the lump is gone."

"What?"

"It's gone. God healed me." Mom was giddy—and believe me, Mom didn't do giddy.

Could it be true? "Mom, what are you saying?"

Her voice gained in decibels. "I'm saying they can't find it. Doctor Herrick had another doctor come in and check me as well. They both agree. It's gone! God healed me! I told you He would."

Just the day before surgery, the lump was large enough to easily feel. Now it had vanished.

If God healed Mom of breast cancer, won't He do that for me, too? I know He can . . . but will He?

A verse came to mind: "Jesus Christ is the same yesterday, today, and forever."[4] *He doesn't change. He healed Dale. He healed Mom. Wouldn't He heal me, too?* A flutter of hope tingled in my stomach.

"Good morning, sweetheart. How are you feeling?" Dale's expansive smile warmed my heart as he ambled into the room, pulling a long-stemmed red rose from behind his back.

"How sweet. Thank you, honey." I smiled as I pulled the fragrant petals to my nose. "Dale, I'm trying to figure some things out. Obviously, it's scary if I really do have cancer. I'm still having trouble believing it. But I've been thinking more about how God answers prayer. I've thought about your amazing recovery from the extensive injuries from the airplane crash. I've also thought about Mom's miracle healing of a malignant tumor.

"You had to work really hard over a period of years, but Mom's miracle was instantaneous. Even though God worked differently in your lives, He still answered your prayers. I know God can answer prayer. I know God can heal. But what I need to know is this. Do you think God will heal *me?*"

"We both know God *can* heal. But knowing God *will* heal is what changes things. Faith comes when we know and believe what God says about healing and is released when we act accordingly. You already know this as well as anyone. But slow down, honey, we don't have to talk about problems or solutions right now. You've been through so much. Wouldn't you rather wait until we get home?"

"No, Dale, I need to talk. If I don't talk about it, I feel like I'll go crazy. I'm trying to believe that God is going to heal me, but then I think about Margie and Nadine. And what about Patty and Jan? They had families, even young children, but they lost their battles with cancer. And then there are Bob and James. These were wonderful people who loved God but died way too young. I know God *can* heal. But I need to know He *will* heal me. How can I think God will do for me what He didn't do for them?"

"I understand, sweetheart. And I'm not trying to minimize the threat. Cancer is the biggest battle we have ever faced. We weren't expecting this blow, and you haven't really had any time to digest it. Don't worry about your faith. I know you. You will rise to the occasion."

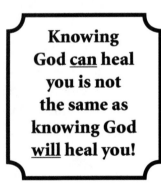

Knowing God <u>can</u> heal you is not the same as knowing God <u>will</u> heal you!

"I guess no one ever expects to have cancer. Right now, I feel panicked. Like I don't have my feet under me. It's like our cockatiel, Toothpick. When you hold her by her body her tiny legs go berserk, flailing in the air trying to find something to grab."

Dale chuckled at the image.

"Well, that's how I feel. I don't have my footing. I know I can find it in God's Word. I just haven't gotten there yet."

"Don't worry. You'll get there; you always have. Now Paula, let me ask you a pointed question. Do you feel angry at God about this?"

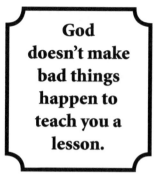

God doesn't make bad things happen to teach you a lesson.

My face contorted in a mixture of emotions. And then it all just sort of poured out of me. "I feel frustrated, Dale. We've given up so much in this world to obey God . . . and now this? Just think about it. We love God and want to serve Him always, but doing what we believed God wanted us to do has cost us everything.

"In the prime of your career, you believed God asked you to surrender your position as an airline pilot to follow Him. As hard as that was, you gave it all up. That was a three million dollar decision, yet I agreed with your choice even though I've second-guessed it a hundred times since. We've led mission teams in dozens of countries at our own expense. Plus, you flew ministers all over the world in our jets at no charge. We've built churches, an orphanage, provided hundreds of thousands of Bibles and gospel tracts. When we needed more money, we'd go back into the business world.

"Even the two jet pilot training companies we built from the ground up—eventually we felt God asked us to surrender them both. I mean, Dale, we've given away houses, jet airplanes, cars, retirement and travel benefits, clout, and a whole lot of money—and security too. We did this willingly in order to follow what we believed God had for us. Now, here we are *again.* Planting a new church out of thin air, trying our best to follow God's plan for our lives. and then BAM . . . to get hit with cancer? What is going on? Why would God let that happen?"

My head collapsed on the pillow in exhaustion. I closed my eyes and squeezed the rose tightly. "Don't get me wrong, Dale. God didn't cause this cancer. I know He doesn't make bad things happen to teach us a lesson. But He certainly allowed it. This is so completely unexpected. It seems totally unfair. I'm not sure I can muster the strength to even fight this battle, let alone win." I shook my head from side to side. Tears trickled down my face. "I'm so tired, Dale. I'm just exhausted."

Dale placed a hand softly on my shoulder. "I know, Paula. It's overwhelming." Wiping a tear from my cheek, he bent and kissed my forehead. "I sure didn't expect this either. I'm so sorry." He looked out the window. I could see the frustration on his face. And then resolve. Whether Dale was trying to convince himself or me, I didn't know, but I was grateful for his encouraging words: "We *will* get through this, Paula. We'll find God's will in this. I promise."

CHAPTER 3

To Believe

≈

*D*r. Anderson eased into the room. I felt fortunate that he was my surgeon. He was well thought of in the community, and my primary physician had made a substantial effort to arrange for me to see him. His pleasant manner and genuine concern made him easy to talk to. I guessed him to be in his mid-50s, though his tall, trim stature belied his age. A full head of sandy-colored hair tinged with silver gave him a distinguished appearance.

"Good morning, you two. How are you feeling, Paula?"

"Hi, Doc."

He smiled as he picked up my chart. "Are you in any pain, Paula?" He matter-of-factly pulled back the bandage on my breast to check the incision.

"Well, right now the physical pain isn't the problem. But my emotions? Not so good."

"That's understandable. This is a big blow for anyone." He replaced the bandage and jotted some notes on my chart.

"Let me ask you, Doc—are you positive my tumor is malignant? Are you completely sure?"

I glanced at Dale. His face tightened. I turned back toward Dr. Anderson. He paused a moment. "Yes, Paula, I'm afraid so. We received the full report from pathology this morning, and it confirms what they told us yesterday. The tumor *is* malignant. You do have cancer."

The room went silent as Dr. Anderson gave us a moment to come to grips with the definitive, unambiguous conclusion from the lab.

It's official. I have to believe it.

I looked at Dale and knew he must have been thinking the same thing. I could tell he was struggling. He seemed suddenly unsteady on his feet. His face was pale. We both gathered ourselves, and I broke the excruciating silence. "Okay, Dr. Anderson, can you tell us what we can expect next?"

"Well, here's the situation. I couldn't get the entire tumor out yesterday. It had spread—like tentacles. I removed the core, but there's still a substantial amount of cancer in your body. I recommend we schedule you for a mastectomy. That means we'll remove your entire breast. At the same time, I'd like to remove some lymph nodes from under your arm to determine how much your cancer has spread. Because of your age and the aggressiveness of this type of cancer, we'll need to get you started on chemotherapy and radiation treatments right away."

Dale interrupted. "What if she doesn't do those things, Doc? What if she just says no to all this? What happens then?"

"Well, as I mentioned, her cancer is very aggressive. If you don't do the treatments, I don't think Paula will be here in three months. Six months maximum." His blue-gray eyes locked onto mine. "In my opinion, you really don't have much choice here."

My hands tightened into fists. "When do we need to do the surgery?"

"As soon as possible. You'll want a little time to find a reconstructive surgeon if you choose to have reconstruction done at the same time. I'd also like to have you meet with the oncologist I work with. I think you'll like him."

"I guess there's no time to waste. I don't want this cancer in my body any longer than necessary."

Dale spoke up again. "Doc, what can Paula do in the meantime to keep the cancer from spreading? If anything will help her, we'll do it."

"Nothing, really. That's why it's so important to get Paula into the chemo and radiation treatments as soon as possible. Why don't we meet in my office on Friday to talk about everything in detail?"

Dale scrunched his face in confusion. "Really? There's nothing she can do? Wow, that's surprising." His eyes widened. "Then . . . I guess we'll see you on Friday." The two shook hands as though some binding agreement had just been reached.

Did I agree? Do I have a choice? Everyone is speaking as if this is normal. Like we're bringing a car in for repairs. But it's my body. My life.

I need to get out of this hospital.

"When do you think I can go home, Doc?"

"You can go home today. Everything looks fine. I'll sign the papers and get you released." Dr. Anderson smiled reassuringly, then turned and left.

Dale sat on the edge of my bed, gently squeezing my toes through the sheet, and looked into my eyes. "Now that you've heard the details from the doctor, how do you feel, honey? What are your thoughts?"

"Gosh, Dale, I don't really know how I feel. I assume I have all the bad news. I just don't know what it all means yet."

"We've just been handed a huge challenge. But if God has

allowed cancer in your life, He'll use it for our good and His glory . . . *if* we do this His way."

"Dale, when you were dealing with all the news from your doctor after the airplane crash, how did you get your faith jump-started?"

"That's a great question, honey. Well, one of the first things I learned was that praying for faith didn't increase my faith. The Bible says, 'Faith comes by hearing, and hearing by the Word of God.'[5] I learned that faith comes from knowing what God says in His Word. The best way, well, the only way to build faith is to read the Bible with an open mind and heart to learn what God says. So I studied the promises of God, trusted them, and released my faith by acting as if that Word were true in my daily life. So faith doesn't come by praying for it. Instead, faith comes by knowing and trusting in God's Word. That's how faith works. But you know this, Paula."

> **If God has allowed cancer in your life, He'll use it for your good and His glory . . . if you do things His way.**

"Then I should do the same thing. When we get home, I need to listen to the audio tapes of Bible promises nonstop so I'm hearing the Word of God constantly. That will help build my faith."

Dale nodded. "That's right, Paula. God hasn't changed. His will is to heal. Through His Word, He'll reveal what you need to do, just as He did for me and as He does for others. It's going to be okay, sweetheart. We'll find God's way through this."

"I'm desperate for that. I need to know what He wants me to do. I realize my course may be different from yours, but I'm sure the principles will be the same. I have to find the path God has for me." Faith doesn't come by praying for it.

"Now that sounds like the Paula I know. You can do this, honey. And I'll be right here with you each step of the way.

It's your body. You're the one with cancer, so it's up to you to make all the final decisions. But we're in this together."

"Thank you, Dale. You know what they say . . . what doesn't kill you makes you stronger. I'm not going to let cancer kill me. I have way too much to live for."

> **Faith doesn't come by praying for it. Faith comes by knowing and trusting in God's Word, then acting on His promises.**

"I completely agree. Hey, why don't I go to the nurses' station and figure out what we need to do to get you out of here this morning? Let's blow this joint."

I smiled. "That sounds great, Dale." He turned to leave. "Dale?"

"Yes, sweetheart?"

"I think I'm ready for a hug—a gentle one, of course." Dale softly embraced me, causing my eyes to fill with unexpected tears. I felt his strength and smiled. Somehow, I knew it would be okay.

Left alone in the room, I reflected more on my circumstances. I'd soon be leaving the hospital to rejoin the outside world. But now I carried in my body a disease called cancer. *Will people be able to tell? Does it show?*

We all die sometime. Is this my time? Is this my way? I've seen dozens of family and close friends succumb to cancer in my short lifetime. What a horrible way to die. Will I die like they did?

I shuddered at the thought.

Death was staring me in the face. Dr. Anderson had said if I didn't do all he recommended, I'd have three to six months. And if he was wrong, death could come even sooner. I remembered the news about Jacqueline Kennedy. She'd been diagnosed with a non-Hodgkin's lymphoma and given five years to live. But she was dead in five months.

Everyone dies, including me—which may be sooner rather than later. I need to be sure about where I'll go when I die. I need to be ready for whatever happens. It's time to revisit my beliefs. My eternal destination depends on knowing the truth.

Everyone has a need to believe in something. Even believing in nothing is believing in something. It seems that God designed us with a "believer" inside.

I need to know the truth. I don't have the luxury to believe something just because I was raised a certain way. I can't afford to play games with religion or traditions or believe something because I like a particular outcome. I have to be certain of the truth. The whole truth . . . the real truth . . . about eternal life.

All through my young life and even more as an adult, I enjoyed reading the Bible. Through extensive study and trying to live out God's Word, I repeatedly experienced the truth of the Bible in my own life. God's Word "proved" itself again and again. The Bible gradually became the only stable truth I could find in this crazy world.

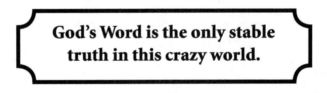

God's Word is the only stable truth in this crazy world.

I thought back to my childhood. As a kid, I felt alone. No matter where I was or how many people surrounded me, I was always lonely. But the loneliness vanished when I invited Jesus into my heart. That was a dramatic moment for me. Never to be lonely again. But it was not just the solution to my loneliness—it was a complete life-changing experience. Something supernatural had happened. More than being changed—I had been transformed.

The details of that experience played back in my mind. I was twelve and in the sixth grade.

Dad was the pastor of a small church in a small town.

Often he'd take a second or even third job to support our family of six.

One night I was helping Dad do janitor work at one of his extra jobs. I loved spending time with him even if I had to empty trashcans and wipe out ashtrays. We'd usually take a break, and he'd buy me a candy bar from a vending machine. That was my favorite time—just Dad and me and no interruptions.

We sat on the floor, backs against the wall. The recent death of a family friend had stirred up questions in me about death and what happens afterward.

"Dad, where will I go when I die? Will I go to heaven?"

He smiled at my innocence. "Well, that depends, Paula. The Bible tells us that to go to heaven one must believe Jesus is God's Son. Do you remember this verse? 'For God so loved the world . . .'? Do you remember the rest of it?"

"For God so loved the world that He gave His only begotten Son, that whoever believes in Him should not perish but have everlasting life. John 3:16."

"Good, honey. That's exactly right."

"Well, I believe that, Dad. I do believe Jesus is the Son of God. Does that mean I get to go to heaven?"

"Well, let me ask you if you remember this verse: 'For all have sinned and fallen short of the glory of God.' That's Romans 3:23."

"Yeah, I've heard that before."

"And what about this one, Paula? 'For the wages of sin is death, but the gift of God is eternal life in Christ Jesus our Lord.'"[6]

"Yeah, I've heard that too."

"That's great, honey, but there's something very important I'd like to ask. Have you asked Jesus to forgive you for your sins? Have you invited Him into your heart?"

"Well, I want to do that, Dad. And if I do, does that mean I get to go to heaven when I die?"

"Yes, it does, Paula. You see Jesus *is* the Son of God. He paid *our* death penalty when He died in *our* place. The Bible says, 'But God demonstrates His own love toward us, in that while we were still sinners, Christ died for us.'[7] And do you remember this one, Paula? 'The blood of Jesus Christ His son cleanses us from all sin'?[8] Do you believe these things, sweetheart?"

"I do, Dad. I really do."

Then Dad quoted a verse I hadn't heard before. "But as many as received Him, to them He gave the right to become children of God, to those who believe in His name."[9] That night Dad led me in prayer and I invited Jesus into my heart. I became a child of God. I also became part of the worldwide family of God spanning generations and have felt an amazing sense of belonging ever since. From that moment on, I knew I would live with God in heaven when my life on earth ends.

> Jesus said, "I am the way, the truth and the life. No one comes to the Father except through Me."
>
> John 14:6

Some memories are so seared into our hearts we carry them to our grave. That decision I made as a twelve-year-old girl helping my dad with his janitor work is one of them.

If this cancer kills me, I am confident I will go to heaven. If I die, I know I'm ready. I know my God is real; I sense His presence every day. He is more real than the ground I stand on.

Simple faith started my journey, but evidence had been building ever since. In Jesus' name, I had seen broken lives restored. Watched hate and anger turn to love and forgiveness. I'd seen drug addicts cured. Marriages healed. I once prayed for a dying woman, her body riddled with cancer, and watched her walk out of hospice—cancer free. A dying friend, in her last breath, awoke from a coma, sat up with a radiant smile, pointed, and whispered, 'Jesus.' My list seemed endless—too many examples to count. Time after time, I'd witnessed the results of God at work.

I'm positive God is real. Heaven is real too. I'll bet my life on it.

Just then Dale came back into the room. "Okay, honey, we're all set. They're going to bring up a wheelchair to take you down and we can leave. Are you ready?"

"Yes, Dale." I smiled. "I'm ready."

CHAPTER 4

Way of Escape

⌒

*L*eaving the hospital was a shock to my system. This was our first summer in the desert and the weather had turned from overcast to blistering hot. In one step I went from a cool, climate-controlled environment into a wall of heat. Air-conditioning isn't a luxury in Palm Desert. It's a life support system. I used to laugh at those supermarket tabloid reports of people walking down the sidewalk and spontaneously combusting, but after one summer in the desert, I no longer laughed. It could happen.

Home at last, I cranked up the air. It felt good to be back in familiar surroundings. With a little imagination, the last two days could have been nothing more than a bad dream.

Dale and I made ourselves comfortable on the couch, cooling down with frosty glasses of iced tea. "Dale, I know you've been spending time at the library looking for answers. What are you learning?"

"We really haven't known anything about what cancer is or where it comes from—or how to combat it. When we learned your diagnosis, I knew it would be vital to have more information, so I've been doing research. You know me—I want to understand everything."

"That's awesome, Dale. I'm so glad you're doing that. You have to tell me everything you're learning."

"Absolutely. This research will take quite a bit of time—there's a lot of information to sift through. But it could save your life, so it's more than worth it."

I grimaced at the reminder of my precarious situation. "What can you tell me so far?"

"Well, I've learned that cancer is basically a group of over a hundred diseases. There are lots of different kinds of cancer but all cancers start when normal cells become damaged and lose their genetic programming. When that happens, they become abnormal cells and reproduce in an uncontrolled manner. In other words, the defective cells duplicate into more defective cells and grow out of control."

My face scrunched up. "What does that mean?"

"Let's start with this." Dale straightened in his seat. "The body is made up of trillions of living cells. These cells have a normal way to grow, divide, and die. Healthy cells are designed by God to function in an orderly fashion. In a healthy person, when a cell becomes damaged or abnormal, the immune system defends the body by surrounding the bad cells with good cells that eliminate the abnormal cells. White blood cells treat abnormal cells like foreign invaders and wipe them out."

"Okay, so this is how a healthy system works. But what happens to this healthy process when somebody gets cancer?"

"Paula, listen to this." Leaning forward, Dale continued. "Everyone has cancer cells in their body. Even babies. But not everyone gets cancer. We all have abnormal and damaged cells. I learned that when someone is diagnosed with cancer, it means the immune system is no longer as effective as it needs to be. The cancer cells are growing faster than they can be eliminated by our white blood cells."

I squirmed in my spot on the couch. "This sounds a lot like biology class, but that was a long time ago. You'll need to remind me how this works, Dale. Can you tell me why these abnormal cells are so deadly?"

"Good question, Paula. In a nutshell, cancer cells invade healthy tissue and drain vital nutrients. And they serve no helpful purpose. They keep duplicating, never die, and eventually overwhelm the immune system."

> **Everyone has cancer cells in their body—but not everyone gets cancer.**

My head cocked. "Hmm, that actually makes sense."

Dale continued. "By the time a tumor is large enough to feel in your body, the cancer cells have been multiplying for a long time. I mean a pinhead-sized tumor usually takes years to develop.

"There's a lot more to learn, Paula, so unless you need me here, I should get back to the library. The obvious questions are . . . what causes cancer and how can a person be cured of cancer. If there are answers, I'm determined to find them. We already know God wants to heal you. We know there are things you can do to build your faith. But in the physical or natural areas that deal with your body, we need to do some fast learning. But first, can I tell you something interesting?"

"Sure, of course."

"Already I've read articles that indicate cancer should never be an automatic death sentence." Dale reached over and took my hand. "Many people have fought back and regained their health. Many have learned how to conquer cancer in the face of horribly overwhelming odds, suggesting cancer can even be reversed—I just don't know how yet. But no matter how bad things get, it is always, *always* too soon to give up hope."

"That sounds good, Dale. I want very much to believe that."

"Honey, I know you want to call the kids and your folks. How about I head back to the library and give you some time to talk to family? I've kept them updated on the basics, but I think they'd rather hear details from you."

"That's a good plan. I really need to give them the news. I've been putting it off, but I can't any longer. I'm sure they're wondering."

Dale grabbed his keys and headed out the door. Now alone, I gathered my thoughts, picked up the phone, and dialed my parents.

Dad answered on the second ring. "Oh, honey, we've been waiting for your call. How are you?"

"I'm fine, Dad, but I have some news that isn't so good." Taking a deep breath, I prepared to dive into the rapids. The phone clicked as Mom picked up the bedroom extension. I swallowed hard. "Mom, Dad, the doctor couldn't remove the entire tumor. It had spread too much. And here's the bad news... it's malignant." My voice broke. "I have cancer."

Stunned silence. Time stopped. Finally, Dad spoke. "Oh, honey. I'm so sorry." I could hear the anguish in his faltering voice. I hurt for both of them.

Mom was quiet. Then, ever the pragmatic parent, asked the obvious. "What are you going to do, Paula?"

Plowing forward, I filled them in on my plans to date. I didn't tell them the whole story. I couldn't burden them with "three to six months." The basics would be enough for now.

Dad sighed long and hard. "Oh, my word."

My parents loved me deeply and even though they lived a ten-hour drive north of us, we were closely connected.

Trying to minimize the threat, I uttered, "I'll be fine. If I'm going to get cancer, this is as good a time as any. I can handle this. Don't you worry—I'll be okay." I hoped they believed me, hoped they bought the false bravado.

We talked about my cancer and about Mom's miracle several years earlier. By the time the call was ending, I sensed Mom and Dad were responding to my crisis exactly as I had hoped.

"Can we pray for you, Paula?"

"That would be nice, Dad. Thanks. I can use all the prayer I can get."

"Dear Lord . . ." Silence. I knew what that meant. Dad sputtered and blew his nose and continued with a shaky voice. He always carried a hankie in his pocket—for good reason. Dad was an old softie. "We ask that You touch Paula and heal her body." Dad paused to wipe his nose again. "Give her and Dale the strength they need to walk through this challenge . . . to face whatever they must face." Dad broke down and could barely finish. "We trust You, Lord. We ask that Your will be done. We pray this in the name of Jesus. Amen." More nose blowing. Emotions were thick and even I could barely keep my shields up.

Mom jumped in. "We love you, honey. If you need anything—I mean anything—we're here for you, okay?" They knew I wasn't telling them everything, but they didn't pry. They knew me. Knew that's the way I wanted it.

We said our goodbyes and I hung up fast. *Why are my hands shaking?* Although I seldom allowed it, I wanted to cry. I longed for Dad and Mom to jump on the next plane and fly down to hold me, hug me, and make it all better. *Paula, you can do this. I can do all things through Christ who strengthens me.*

Despite my claims that everything would be okay, tears fell and I couldn't stop them. Once again, I failed miserably to brace up the dam. This time it completely crumbled and I was in danger of being swept away.

Thank goodness Dale knows how bad everything is. He'll go through this with me. Together we'll find God's will. I knew how hard this was for Dale. So far, he had put on a brave front, but there were telltale signs of his struggle.

There was another person I needed to call—my sister. Marna and I were close. Telling her I had cancer would be difficult; she wouldn't let me sidestep things the way Dad and Mom had. Wiping my eyes, I dialed her number.

The call with Dad and Mom helped me maneuver through the conversation with my sister. I skirted the details, giving her just enough to satisfy. Discussing my cancer, even with those I loved, was barely possible.

Finally, I called our two children, Eric and Kara. Dale had been keeping them informed at every turn, but I knew they still wanted to hear my voice. I couldn't wait to talk to each of them. I shared some details and did my best to answer their questions about my cancer. They were both very supportive and I felt enormously blessed to be loved so much.

Sinking into an overstuffed chair, I dropped my face in both hands. *Whew! That was hard.* It was a blessing to have family who loved me and would be there when I needed them. But with or without family, I knew I belonged to God. He was the One who had what I needed. *Only God can walk me safely through this storm.* Although my head knew He would do this, my heart hadn't yet made it to that higher ground.

Reaching for my Bible on the nightstand, I pleaded, "Lord, I need to hear from You right now. Please tell me what to do. Speak to me from Your Word, Father." My quiet prayer embodied my desperate need and carried all my hopes toward heaven.

Hunched over my Bible, I combed through the pages for answers. On and on I read, filled with anticipation. *Lord, I need something from You.* Verse after verse, I pressed on. Suddenly my heart gave a small lurch. *What? What did that say?* I read it again, my heart pounding in my chest. *Is this it? Is this for me?*

I read the verse aloud. "God will not tempt you beyond

that which you are able to endure without making a way of escape."[10] I read the verse again. And again. *Without making a way of escape? God won't tempt me or test me beyond my ability without making a way of escape? Is that what it means?* Memorizing the chapter and verse, I reached for my pen and underlined the words.

Searching the footnotes for more understanding, I discovered that in the original text, the word *tempt* actually meant "to allow trial or testing." His Word promised a way through the testing to a safe landing place. God would not allow any trial to be more than I could handle without showing me my way of escape.

Reading the entire chapter again, I made sure I understood the context of the words. Next I focused on the verse and read it over and over. *Is this God's promise for me?* My heart leaped with hope each time I reviewed the sacred words. *Yes, this must be for me . . . for my battle with cancer. This promise is for me—for right now!*

"God will not tempt you beyond that which you are able to endure without making a way of escape."

1 Corinthians 10:13

God had faithfully spoken to me this way many times in the past. When I found scripture in the Bible that stirred my heart, and then acted upon it in faith, it had proved to be my answer every time. But then, it had never been cancer before.

I wonder if God really will give me a "way of escape." If so, will I be healed? What will He use to bring healing? A miracle? The medical system? Surgery, chemo, and radiation? Or does He have something else in mind? I smiled at the possibility.

47

The fear that had been making its home in the pit of my stomach suddenly felt uprooted. Something more powerful was vying for position. Faith had been sparked by a Bible promise—a personal promise. Direct from God to me.

CHAPTER 5

The Cancer Club

⌇

"*T*'ll meet you in the doctor's office, okay?" Dale let me out and sped off to park the car.

I took the elevator to Dr. Anderson's office, noticing the faint smell of disinfectant in the air.

Is this my new life? Hospitals, medical tests, doctor appointments?

In Dr. Anderson's waiting area, I grabbed a pair of vacant seats next to an attractive black woman and introduced myself. "Hello. My name's Paula. Are you a patient?"

"Hi. I'm Jada. Yes, I'm here to see Dr. Anderson."

"Me too. It looks like we could be here a while." Lowering my voice and leaning closer, "Jada, do you think everyone here has cancer?"

She nodded. "Probably. I just started my second round of chemo."

"Oh, wow, that must be terribly difficult." *Second round? I haven't even considered that possibility.* "I'm supposed to start chemo soon and I'm not looking forward to it. Can you tell me what it's like?"

"Believe me, girl, it's no fun. I can tell you that much. I found out I had breast cancer almost three years ago and thought I had beat it with the first round of chemo and radiation. But recently I found another lump and have to start the whole routine again."

"That's terrible. Jada, I'm so sorry. What does that mean?"

"Well, short and simple, it means either they didn't get it all the first time or I just got cancer again." Anxiety was written all over her face. "I can't tell what good the darn chemo did and now they tell me I have to get the treatments again. I'm dreading it." Fear was swimming in Jada's eyes as she leaned in and whispered, "You know, my cousin was having chemo last year and the dosage they gave him was too high. He died right in the chair."

My mouth dropped wide open. *How could something that's supposed to help you, kill you? And how could cancer come back after treatment?* My nightmare just got a lot scarier.

Jada's voice strained. "Last time, I only had a lumpectomy 'cause the lump was small. But this time they removed my entire breast. Plus the chemo and radiation makes ya so darn sick. It's no life, Paula. It's a living nightmare." Her eyes bore into me with a look that said, *I wouldn't wish cancer on my worst enemy.*

I sighed. "I never considered getting cancer twice or that chemo was so dangerous."

"Last time it took forever to get my strength back and feel normal again."

Could that be me next year . . . or the year after that?

By then, Dale had entered the waiting area and had taken the seat next to mine. He had overheard some of Jada's remarks and appeared to be reeling from them. But Dale couldn't pass up the opportunity to gather more data, especially direct, firsthand information. He introduced himself to Jada and the two began talking while I scanned the room.

A dozen or so people were seated, waiting. *How many of these people are having chemo? It must be safe or so many wouldn't do it . . . would they?* I couldn't help but notice several patients with obvious hair loss. Some were wearing wigs. Some were wearing scarves. I turned and eyed Jada's soft, sleek bob. It was beautiful. *I wonder if . . .*

"It's a wig," she smiled, as if reading my thoughts.

"Well, it looks great. I guess I'll need to do some shopping of my own." *I'll probably lose my hair from chemo.* My hair was long and blonde. Dale loved it. Heck, I liked it, too.

"Say, you mentioned you're just starting the process. If I can help, I'd be happy to." Jada pulled a piece of paper from her purse and scribbled on it. "Here's my phone number. Talking to others who understand what you're going through can help."

"That would be wonderful." I quickly jotted down my phone number and handed it to her. "Can I ask where you got your wig? It's lovely and so natural."

Gently patting her hair, she beamed. "Well, thank you. It does help to feel like I look nice—and no one can tell there's a problem." She wrote down the names of a couple of shops in the area.

"Jada Johnson!" the nurse summoned.

There is still so much I'd like to ask her . . .

The three of us exchanged warm goodbyes. Wearing a thousand-watt smile, Jada turned and hugged me. With her arms around me, she whispered, "Call me. You're going to need my advice." She chuckled.

I looked into her deep brown eyes and smiled back. "I will. Definitely. And thank you, Jada."

Dale softly grasped Jada's hand and squeezed. "And, Jada, if *you* need anything, we're here for you too. Okay?"

Choking up, Jada nodded, then turned and soon disappeared from view.

Oh, she's such a sweetheart. I really like her. But cancer twice! I can't believe she is going through this a second time. Does that really happen to people?

Our brief conversation with Jada had added to our list of questions. Dale and I exchanged wondering looks.

"Paula Black!" *Now it's my turn.*

Dale and I trailed the nurse to the examination room. It seemed clear the staff had their system down to a science. Another day, different people. *What happened to the patients who came through here last month? Last year? Where are they now? How many are still alive?*

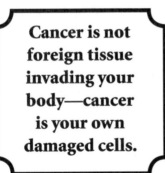

Cancer is not foreign tissue invading your body—cancer is your own damaged cells.

I sat on the examination table while Dale plunked down in the corner chair. The room was small but pleasant. I knew the routine. We'd have to wait a while for the doctor to show up.

"Dale, it looks like we have some time. What else have you learned about cancer that might help us?"

"Quite a bit, actually. It's interesting stuff. Did you know that normal cells can't invade other tissues in the body? But cancer cells can. You see, when DNA-damaged cells invade other areas of the body, they can multiply and group together. That's what forms a tumor."

"So are you saying that cancer isn't some foreign tissue? Cancer is our own damaged cells?"

"Yes, that's right. All forms of cancer have a couple of things in common. First, they consist of abnormal cells that reproduce themselves, and, second, instead of dying, they grow out of control and cause all types of damage. I also learned that cancer cells can travel to other parts of the body in two different ways—in the blood stream or through the lymph system. And once they spread to another area, they usually grow and form new tumors. Do you know what that's called?"

"The doctor calls that metastasis. Is that right?"

"Exactly. It's just a fancy word that means the cancer has spread to another area."

"Dale, the doctor is talking about taking out some of my lymph nodes. Do you know what the value of that is? And what are they, anyway?"

"As a matter of fact, I did learn about that. The lymph network is a lot like the veins that carry blood through the body. But instead of carrying blood, it carries clear watery fluid called lymph. Lymph fluid carries oxygen and other nutrients to the cells. The fluid also contains white blood cells that help fight infections. The lymph nodes are like tiny filters that remove harmful substances in the fluid and contain immune cells that attack and destroy germs. Your lymph network is a vital part of your immune system."

"Then why does the doctor want to remove some of my lymph nodes? If they're part of my immune system, shouldn't I keep all of them?"

"Well, since cancer cells are spread by either the blood or lymph fluid, the doctor can usually determine whether cancer has spread by checking if it is in the lymph nodes nearest the tumor."

"Okay, that explains why the doctor wants to remove some of my lymph nodes. So it really doesn't do anything except give him information. But if cancer does spread to another area, does it become a different type of cancer?"

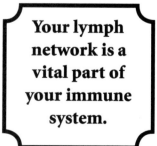

Your lymph network is a vital part of your immune system.

"No. The type of cancer is named for the place it started. For example, in your case, Paula, breast cancer. If it spreads to the liver, it is called metastatic breast cancer. It's not called liver cancer. Remember the pilot we worked with—Bill? He had prostate cancer. Even though it spread to his bones, when he died it was determined that he died of prostate cancer because that's where it originated."

"That makes sense in a weird sort of way. No one dies from a tumor in their breast, yet people die of breast cancer all the time. Now I get it. They actually die from cancer cells that have spread to another area and formed new tumors. I remember the doctor saying that the most common places for breast cancer to spread to were the bone, brain, liver, and lungs."

"Yes. That's right. And different kinds of cancers behave differently. If the cancer's in the blood, like lymphoma, it behaves one way; if it's in the bones, it behaves differently than in the liver. Basically, we're still talking about the same thing though—cells that are damaged and multiply and don't die, no matter what name you give them."

"Dale, what about a tumor that's benign?"

"Yeah, not all tumors are malignant. But even benign tumors can cause problems if they grow large enough and press on healthy organs and tissues. The thing about a benign tumor is that the cells don't grow into or invade other tissues. They also can't spread to other parts of the body. So a benign tumor is usually not life threatening. Now . . . let me ask you if you're ready for some shocking stats."

"Sure. Hit me with 'em. I need to know everything you know."

"Listen to this, Paula. According to the American Cancer Society, half of all men and one third of all women in the United States will develop cancer in their lifetime."

"Are you kidding me? Did I hear you right?"

"Yep. Look Paula, I wrote this down. I could hardly believe

it myself. Let me get my notes." Dale unfolded three pieces of paper he had pulled from his pocket. "Okay, see for yourself."

I looked over his notes. Approximately 1,660,290[11] new cancer cases were expected to be diagnosed that year. That totals 4,548 people per day.

"Oh, my goodness. Then how many people will die from it?"

"According to the American Cancer Society, about 580,350[12] Americans are expected to die of cancer this year alone. That's an average of fifteen-hundred and ninety people a day. The ACS's own numbers tell us that thirty-five percent of those diagnosed will die. Cancer is the second leading cause of death in the U.S., exceeded only by heart disease."

"So if I look around at the people in my world, half of the men and a third of the women will deal with cancer sometime. Wow! But then if you stop and think about it, my mom had cancer and now I have it—that's two-thirds of the women in my family. And Mom, her brother, and two of her sisters had cancer. That's four-fifths of her siblings. Half of them died of their cancer. And you're saying about sixteen hundred die every day in the U.S.? That's a lot of cancer."

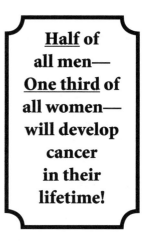

Half of all men— **One third** of all women— will develop cancer in their lifetime!

"If you look at this other page, Paula, you're going to be shocked even more. . . ."

Our conversation was sidelined as the doctor stepped into the room. Dale quickly stuffed his notes back into his pocket.

Dr. Anderson had a way of making cancer seem like a simple cold or the flu—something manageable. The first time we met, he told me his mother was dealing with breast cancer too. As if it were something everyone had to cope with, as if it were not that big a deal. There were no telltale signs that he was worried—at least none I could see. I wondered how his mother was doing but didn't have the guts to ask.

"How are you doing today, Paula?"

"Okay, I guess."

"Well, as I mentioned to you in the hospital, we need to schedule another surgery. I'm recommending a radical mastectomy."

I wanted to ask if there was any other choice. An easier way out. But I already knew the answer. "When, doc?"

"As soon as we can. How would next Wednesday work?"

I turned toward Dale. I needed backup. "What do you think, honey?"

"That'll work for me. But it's your decision, Paula. Obviously, we should get the rest of the cancer out as soon as possible . . . shouldn't we?"

The ball was back in my court. "Sure. Of course we should." *I want the cancer out. But it's going to cost me part of my body. And not just any part. My tonsils I could do without, but my breast? That's different. It will change everything.* I wanted to scream. Somehow I managed to hold it together and heard myself say, "Okay, doc. Let's schedule it for next Wednesday."

"Great." Dr. Anderson flashed his signature smile. *I'm glad someone is pleased.* "Same routine, nothing to eat or drink after midnight on Tuesday. I'll see you both at the hospital at 6:30 A.M. I'd also like you to visit Dr. Marcus before the surgery. He's the oncologist I told you about. Here's his information— you should call right away to make an appointment."

After some final pleasantries, Dr. Anderson hurried off to his next patient.

Later that day I called to schedule an appointment with the oncologist. But what I really wanted was to talk to people who had gone through what I was about to go through—women who had had breast cancer. I needed more answers. The short talk with Jada had helped. If I could find others like her, maybe I could piece together a plan I'd feel good about.

I shared my idea with my parents, and Dad put me in touch with Sherry, a woman in his office who had been diagnosed with breast cancer five years earlier. Sherry had had her breast removed and had gone through a full round of chemo and radiation. Three years later they found cancer in her other breast. She had to repeat the entire course of action. . . . Twice. *That's two people I've talked to who had cancer twice.*

"Sherry," I asked her, "if you had to do the entire process again, would you do anything different?"

She took her time responding, telling me the reasons behind all her decisions. Her answers gave me food for thought. I asked how she was doing now, two years after her second bout with cancer. "Good. I'm feeling pretty healthy again. I hope, now that I have no breasts, the threat is over."

Speaking with Sherry was helpful, but I wanted more. Donna, the sister of a woman I worked with, had breast cancer and agreed to talk to me. I was surprised to discover that people with cancer were usually willing, even eager, to talk about it. I found that it was constantly on their minds, but they didn't seem to feel free to talk openly unless someone asked them. My questions gave release to a tension that was always present. Now that I had cancer, I was an initiated member of the club.

Picking up the phone, I called Donna. She candidly shared her journey from the day she learned she had cancer until the present. Donna had an open, expressive personality and I found my emotions running the gamut as she related her experience. As I would discover with all the women I would talk to, there were countless twists and turns to their stories, countless losses and victories. Life would never be the same for these women. Once independent and full of life, they were now sidelined and challenged in ways I had never considered.

"Donna, can I ask you what you like about the choices you made and what you wish you had done differently?"

"Sure, Paula. Well, I did everything. They removed my breast and some lymph nodes, and then I endured chemotherapy and radiation. I had reconstruction on my breast, so I didn't have to deal with a prosthetic."

"Are you glad you did that?"

"Yes, I am. I would do it again if I had to."

"What about the chemo and radiation?"

"Well, the chemo made me ever so sick and I lost my hair. I decided I had to do it because the cancer was in my lymph nodes and my doctor was afraid it had already spread. The radiation made me extremely tired. I couldn't seem to do anything while I was taking the treatments. Unfortunately, I'm still sensitive and have some residual pain. I don't know if that area will ever feel normal."

"Would you do chemo and radiation again if you had it to do over?"

"I guess so. The doctor thought it was necessary and I wanted to get rid of the cancer, so I did whatever he recommended."

"Is the cancer gone now?"

"Well, it seems to be. My last checkup showed no tumors, so I'm hoping everything I did worked out. I'm keeping my fingers crossed."

"I hope so too, Donna. Thank you for being so open." I had a new friend. And a weird sense of belonging to this "cancer club" I had involuntarily joined.

I spoke to five women in all. Five women who had journeyed across the waters I was about to sail. They were all alive and seemingly cancer free. All except Jada, who was fighting cancer for the second time, but she was in treatment and everyone was hopeful.

My investigation had turned up some interesting facts. Information that revealed the intense struggles that can accompany cancer, as well as choices I hadn't considered before.

Lying on the couch and staring at the ceiling, I replayed the conversations with my five new friends. Their personal struggles broke my heart . . . in places I didn't know could break.

CHAPTER 6

Cracking Open
Pandora's Box

⤳

My brain was on overload again. I had spent two days talking to my five new friends and had gathered an avalanche of information. Dale and I sat up long into the night trying to make sense of it all. One particular thought relentlessly persisted. Two of the five women had a recurrence of cancer. That's a pretty high percentage. And who was to say cancer wouldn't return in one or more of the other three? It started to become clear to us that the medical industry had created a cancer conveyor belt.

I was on it, with no apparent exit.

Walking into the oncologist's office the next morning, we were greeted warmly by Dr. Marcus. The place was empty of people except for the doctor and his staff. With our early morning appointment, we'd obviously beaten the crowd.

Dr. Marcus laid out my particular needs and recommended treatments. Then, a tour. Lucy, the doctor's assistant, escorted us into the patient treatment area—an inviting large open space with high ceilings and lots of light. Multiple high-back lounge chairs, each equipped with a set of headphones, were arranged in intimate groupings. Several faced TVs while others aimed at windows overlooking lush landscaping. Lucy explained how patients can listen to music, watch TV, or just shut out the noise.

She was a gracious host with ready answers. Politely, she asked, "Do you have any questions I can answer for you?"

Dale, always the joker and consummate connoisseur of old movie and TV lines, interrupted in a decent Desi Arnaz accent. "Lucy, you got some real 'esplainin' to do."

I turned and punched his arm. "Come on, Dale, be serious."

Lucy grinned. Ignoring Dale, she pointed to one of the recliners. "Why don't you try out one of the chairs, Paula?"

"Sure, thanks." I sank into the cushioned armchair and pulled up the footrest. The chairs were indeed comfortable. *They would have to be if people sit here for hours at a time.* I eyed the metal IV dispensers pushed up against the wall. The unspoken harsh reality stormed back in. *You don't get the comfortable chair without the chemicals that ravage your body.*

Lucy saw my gaze and confirmed my thoughts. "Your first time will take longer because we dispense the chemicals slower to see how you tolerate them. After that, if you've handled it okay, the other sessions won't take as long."

Redirecting us toward something more pleasant, Lucy pointed out the small library in the corner where an enticing selection of books and magazines were neatly arranged. "Many like to read while they receive their treatments. Others actually sleep. And Dale, you can come in and sit with Paula if you'd like to."

"Yes, definitely. We're in this together." Always the inquiring mind, Dale asked, "What are the chemicals in the chemo and how strong a dosage will Paula receive?"

"Dr. Marcus will answer any of your treatment questions," she replied.

We concluded our tour just as the first several patients wandered in. Winding out of the parking lot, Dale's voice broke the silence. "Well, Paula, what did you think?"

"I liked Dr. Marcus and his staff. They were all very pleasant." *Keep talking before he asks another question.* "The chairs were comfortable. Did you sit in one?" His expression said it all. He knew I was deflecting.

"Okay, Paula. Seriously. How are you feeling about the chemotherapy?"

Don't want to talk about it! This can't be my life. But Dale knew that, deep down, I needed to discuss it, and I was grateful he cared enough to force the issue.

Panic and desperation collided as I opened my mouth, allowing my thoughts to spill out. "I can't believe this is my world now. I don't want to do this, but I don't feel like I have a choice. Do I? Can I say I'm not going to do it?" The words continued gushing forth. "I mean, who in their right mind— no matter how nice the furnishings and staff are—voluntarily sits for hours while chemicals that make them sick and lose their hair are pumped through their body? Why would I do that? Why would anybody do that? How can the doctors want me to do that?" I could feel my face flush red as my eyes filled with tears.

"Did you see those patients?" I continued. "Am I just another one of them? They looked like they were dying. At least two of them did."

"Paula, I know all this is overwhelming, but let's look at it for what it is. We haven't committed to chemo yet—you still have choices. Let's just think about what we learned this morning and let it simmer for a few days. We don't have to decide until after the surgery. Let's just share our thoughts without making a decision. How does that sound?"

Whoosh. I let out the breath I didn't know I had been holding. My chest relaxed for the first time in an hour. "You're right. I don't have to decide right now. And maybe I don't even have to do chemo. I need more time to deal with everything."

"Good. We'll pray about it and try to find out what God wants you to do. He has an opinion, you know."

"Of course, He does," I replied with a grin. "If I do this His way, there's no reason to freak out, right?"

Dale smiled. "That's right, Paula. How about we do something that's been on our list that's fun?"

"Fun? What's that?" We both chuckled. "What is on our 'to do' list that's fun?"

"Let's go check out those wig shops. Then how about I take you to lunch at that restaurant you've been wanting to try on El Paseo Drive?"

That could be fun. We parked the car and enjoyed a leisurely stroll to the first shop on our list. Assisted by a pleasant saleslady, I tried on a variety of styles and colors, morphing into a different personality with each one. The flirtatious blonde. The aggressive redhead. Then approaching Dale, wearing the look of "the sultry brunette," I innocently asked, "What do you think of this one?"

With a greasy grin, Dale replied in jest. "Louis, I think this is the beginning of a beautiful friendship."

I grinned. "No come on, be serious. Which of the wigs do you like most?"

Holding a ramrod-straight pose and chewing on a toothpick, Dale shot back, "Frankly, my dear, I don't give a darn."

"Good grief. Can't I ask a simple question?" We both laughed.

My spirits lifted as I persisted in pushing cancer from my mind. I knew Dale needed the reprieve as much as I did.

Laughter *is* good medicine, and we were both creating a small but helpful dose of it as I proceeded to turn some lovely bright-colored scarves into something fashionable. But my loops and knots resembled a multi-scarf pile-up more than style. We doubled over again. Shopping *was* helping.

> **It isn't normal to cut out part of my body . . . lose my hair . . . or get sick and exhausted while trying to get well. How can I get better by getting sicker first?**

Eventually the thoughts our outing had held at bay began to strong-arm their way back in. I turned to Dale. "Do you remember hearing Dr. Marcus say I could lose my hair from either the chemo or the radiation? So even if I don't do chemo, I still may need a wig. It's a good excuse to cut my hair really short. I've thought about doing that before but never had the guts. It could be fun. What do you think?"

Dale answered but I suddenly found myself distracted, watching our saleslady and other store employees scurrying around to assist customers. *Everyone in the business of cancer, from the doctors and nurses to the salespeople in the shops, seems to know just how to handle me. Do they go through some special training to make everything seem pleasant and natural?* Our saleslady knew just what to say and how to reassure me. She had me nearly convinced that buying a wig and scarves for a head about to be stripped of hair was the most normal thing in the world.

Nothing about this is normal. It sure isn't normal to cut out part of my body . . . or lose my hair . . . or get sick and exhausted while trying to get well. How can I get better by getting sicker first?

Dale sensed my tension rising. "Let's head to the restaurant before it gets busy. You know I don't do lines," he snickered.

Leaving the shop, we walked briskly to the restaurant and settled into a comfortable booth next to a window. There were more boutiques in this shopper's paradise than anyone could visit in a day. As we sat, I enjoyed watching the people pass by laden with their newfound treasures.

"How are you feeling, Paula?" Dale reached across the table and took hold of my hand.

"You sure ask me that a lot these days," I chuckled. "But to answer your question, I'm overwhelmed—again. I'm sorry I'm such an emotional mess lately, but everything is a contradiction."

"What do you mean?"

"Well, you've seen it. Everywhere we've been today, people were pleasant. The offices and oncology areas were bright and inviting. The wig shops were fun and the salespeople easy to work with. But at the root of all this pleasantness is the ugliness of cancer. I appreciate all the 'nice' on one hand but feel deceived on the other. Does that make any sense?"

"Of course it does, Paula."

As we waited for our server, we made small talk, revisiting fond memories from our past. We recounted some of our family trips, which, of course, brought up our annual vacations spent houseboating on Lake Powell, complete with Jet Skiing, waterskiing, hiking, and—my favorite—fishing. We replayed our various trips to Israel and a few of our mission trips to Guatemala, Ecuador, and Peru. Our life had been full of living and giving—full of unforgettable memories.

"Let's plan a vacation for next year," Dale stated matter-of-factly. "We need to focus on your future. There is still a lot of life for you to live, Paula."

"That's true. I need to remember that, Dale."

A twenty-something waitress with short jet-black hair arrived. "Hi, my name is Nicole and I'll be your server. May I get you something to drink from the bar to get you started?"

Without missing a beat, Dale lowered his voice and responded in jest, "Bond. James Bond. Shaken and not stirred please. And Miss Moneypenny? What would you like, dear?"

I slapped Dale on the arm. "Don't mind him, Nicole. We'd love two iced teas please." I shook my head and grinned across the table as she scurried away smiling.

Dale defended his antics. "I thought we were supposed to be having fun."

Eventually—inevitably—our conversation led back to the cancer. "Paula, now that we've had a little break, what are your thoughts about the surgery and the chemo . . . and losing your hair?"

"It's too hard to think about the whole picture. The only way I know to deal with the issues is to take them one by one. But amid all the confusion, I have this wonderful promise from God—a way of escape. That's the only thing giving me some peace and hope right now. What do you think, Dale?"

"Until God shows us another way, I think we should consider everything the doctor recommends, at least at this point. But let's keep praying. We need to stay expectant. And we need to continue doing our own research, honey. Big time."

"Of course, Dale. I'll keep praying and asking God to reveal something more—if there is more. But I think we're doing what we need to be doing, at least for now. And because of the scripture God gave me, I believe I will eventually be free of cancer. He *will* give me a way of escape. But speaking of research, what else have you learned? You've sure been spending a lot of time at the library and studying the books you brought home."

"Yes, I have, and it's paying off too. Though I have learned a lot, I feel like it's only the tip of the iceberg. There's so much more to learn. Paula, are you ready for some very disturbing information? In preparation for the oncology appointment, I did some research on chemotherapy. And what I found is really upsetting me. This is not easy to share, sweetheart. Is now a good time?"

"Go ahead, Dale. I'm always ready. I need to know everything you're learning."

Looking away, he paused. Then his eyes riveted onto mine. "Chemotherapy is the use of highly dangerous toxins that are administered into the body to kill cancer cells. Because these chemicals are so powerful, they can kill the patient if the dosage is not carefully monitored. Paula, these drugs were initially derived from the nitrogen mustard gas experiments during World War I and World War II. These poisons—and that's exactly what they are—kill *all* fast-growing cells. Well, since cancer cells are fast growing, some genius decided to try these chemicals on cancer. They kill the cancer cells all right, but they kill good cells too. Paula, that's why people lose their hair. Hair cells are fast growing."

"Wow. Dale, that's difficult to believe. Why would anyone use poison to treat cancer? Are you sure about that?"

Nodding, Dale took a long sip of iced tea. "Yes, I am completely sure. And the trick with chemo, from a doctor's perspective, is to give just enough dosage to kill most of the cancer cells but not enough to kill the patient."

I recoiled. "What?"

"Yep. You see, if the doctor uses enough chemo toxins to kill *all* the cancer cells, the patient will die. Paula, this is happening all across our country every day."

"Is that what happened to Jada's cousin? The guy who died right in the chemotherapy chair?"

"Yes, most likely." Dale pulled out another piece of paper from his back pocket. "I'm going to have to make a notebook of all this stuff. Let me read this to you, Paula. Dr. Alan Levin says, '. . . chemotherapy does not work for the majority of cancers.' And 'Most cancer chemotherapy studies consider patients who die of drug toxicity as "unevaluable." These deaths are not factored into the survival statistics.'[13] Can you believe that? When I read that, it stopped me in my tracks. Honey, these are toxic, poisonous chemicals that can kill all life."

"And the doctors are putting this stuff into sick people?" I was stunned. "Then why would anyone use chemotherapy? How can this be the standard treatment for cancer in the first place? This is really confusing. Something doesn't make sense."

"No kidding. Paula, I know this is hard to swallow. Believe me, I wouldn't put a lot of credence in my research about chemo killing patients before the cancer does if it were just one source. But there are a lot of qualified professionals saying the same thing about these toxic treatments."

"What are your conclusions about all the things you're sharing, Dale?"

Leaning back in his seat and slowly exhaling, Dale replied, "I'm trying to sort it out." He took a slow sip of tea before continuing. "But there's another important component to all this. Let's talk about God in this process of using toxic poisons for treating cancer, or any disease for that matter. Does this sound like the God of the Bible? It doesn't sound like the God I know. It's impossible for me to believe God works this way. I can't accept that He would violate His own design by using a substance so unnatural, dangerous, and damaging as a way to heal His creation. There

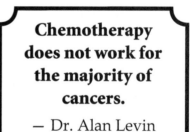

Chemotherapy does not work for the majority of cancers.

— Dr. Alan Levin

is something horribly wrong about chemotherapy, but until I researched this information, I hardly questioned any of it."

"Me neither." Looking out the window, I paused to contemplate. "Well, what about radiation?"

"So far I see nothing but problems with radiation too. I read about a cancer expert who said treating cancer with radiation therapy was like fighting a carpet fire with a rifle.[14] It's the wrong weapon. Furthermore, radiation does a lot of damage to the tens of thousands of good healthy cells trying to fight off disease in the patient's body. In the process of irradiating the cancer tissue, good tissues are obliterated.

"I mean, Paula, the books I'm reading are sending up huge red flags. I'm highly concerned. But keep in mind, I'm not finished yet. I need more time to study, more time to pray and to give you all the variables. I am aware that your life depends on you getting all information correctly and accurately . . . the first time. And I know you need it fast."

"Wow. Dale, my mind is going crazy. I believe you, but I have trouble coming to grips with the fact that Dr. Anderson would recommend these treatments if they were that bad. And how could the entire medical system have it wrong? I'm not ready to throw out the medical protocol based on the comments of a few doctors and supposed experts. I need more information. At the same time, I'm now very wary. So please, keep doing your research. I have to decide what I'm going to do, and I need all the facts. I have to be sure.

"I need some good news. Can you tell me about cancer statistics, Dale? How many people are getting cured? That's what I'm really interested in."

Before Dale could respond, Nicole arrived with our food, halting the conversation. The focus diverted to our meal for several minutes.

Placing a napkin across my lap and pouring some dressing on my salad, I picked up my last question. "What about those statistics, Dale? I really want to hear some good news."

Quickly swallowing his first bite of sandwich, Dale replied. "Paula, it's weird, but I can hardly find any solid stats on that. I haven't wanted to tell you because I'm still researching, but I am having a very hard time finding solid data when it comes to cancer cure rates."

"Really? Why wouldn't you be able to find that kind of information? It's what everyone with cancer wants to know."

"True. But so far, I'm finding very little about rates of people being cured. However, I did find a strange phenomenon."

"And what's that?"

"When I research the American Cancer Society or the National Cancer Institute or any of the other reporting organizations, it looks like I'm reading the exact same material. You know, like they all use the exact same data from the same author. I mean even the wording is almost the same, word for word. What's that all about? That has me puzzled."

"Hmm . . . interesting. Back to the statistics, Dale. Have you found *any* stats at all for cancer cure rates?"

"Paula, this whole thing about cure rates has to be broken down and dissected. I mean, *cancer cure* has to be defined. And talk about loosey-goosey. What I'm finding is strange, even weird."

"Talk about weird."

Dale flashed a smile. "Okay, look. To start with, a person is considered 'cured of cancer' if they don't die within five years of diagnosis. That ain't no cure, baby. If a person dies five years and one day after their diagnosis, that person is statistically still considered cured. Can you believe that? It makes no sense. And it's misleading."

Selecting a page from his papers, Dale continued. "Here's a document I copied. It reflects a study conducted by the Department of Radiation Oncology at a leading cancer center.

"What? That's ridiculous. The cure rate has to be higher than that. What are they referring to?"

Dale sorted through his pages, flattening them with his hand. He had made a copy of a previous issue of *Clinical Oncology.* "Look at this chart, Paula. Here's how it works. This study shows the actual impact of chemotherapy on adults. I've had to do a little sifting and filtering, but chemotherapy as a cancer cure is pathetic. I was expecting a rate of fifty percent or more. Isn't that about what you were thinking?"

"Sure, about half of the people—at least. That's what I would think."

"Right. Well get this. Oh, by the way, I would also have thought that *cancer cure* would mean that the cancer never came back in the patient's lifetime. Right? Wrong. Again, in this report they state that the patient is cured if they do not die within five years."

"These statistics are making me pretty nervous, Dale. I mean, I knew if a person lived for five years after diagnosis, they were considered 'a survivor.' But I didn't realize that's how they were defining 'cured.'"

"Look at this chart, Paula. Can you believe these examples?" For the next several minutes, I studied the chart Dale had placed in front of me. Solid statistics showed that chemotherapy helped less than two percent of colon cancer patients survive for five years. For people with stomach cancer, less than one percent were helped with chemotherapy.

"This is horrible, Dale. I can hardly believe these numbers."

"Well, check this out. Those with pancreatic cancer . . . are you ready for this? Zero percent. That means that according to this study, not one person with pancreatic cancer was helped by chemotherapy; none survived even five years. Melanoma? Also zero percent. Uterine cancer: zero percent. Prostate cancer: zero percent. Non-Hodgkin's lymphoma, a little better, but still less than twelve percent lived for five years. These are just a few examples, Paula. When you put them all together, the bottom line is this: According to this report, chemotherapy helped an average of less than three percent of the cancer patients survive to five years. Is this what you expected to hear? Does that surprise you? It shocks me."

"I am totally stunned! I had no idea the numbers were that

dismal. This is really scaring me, Dale. Chemotherapy barely works. Why should I poison my body for odds *that* terrible? Plus, how much *new* damage does the chemo do?"

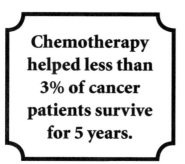

Chemotherapy helped less than 3% of cancer patients survive for 5 years.

"I know, Paula, I know. There's something very strange going on, that's for sure. I've learned so much, but what I've discovered thus far has brought up more questions than answers. Obviously, I have a lot more research to do."

"Thanks, Dale. You know I appreciate all you're doing and learning, even if what you're finding is unsettling. For now, I'm still trusting God and believing He's going to heal me or show us our way through, or both. The verse about God making a way of escape is giving me hope."

"That's wonderful. I'm believing for that too, honey. But as you know, when we use God's Word for direction, we use the culmination of His Word, not just one verse. Remember the Bible says the 'sum of His word is truth.'[15] Right? We have to make sure nothing we're thinking of doing violates any part of God's Word and that what we're believing is found throughout the Bible, not in just one isolated verse."

"Absolutely, Dale. Of course, that's right."

"It's comforting to know we don't have to depend on our own strength and wisdom in a situation as serious as this. Or count on statistics and medical facts. God offers us His wisdom, which is superior to anything this world has to offer. But this is still unbelievably difficult to go through and I'd give almost anything if you . . . we . . . didn't have to."

Dale's tender voice calmed me as it melted my heart. "It will be okay, Paula. Remember all the things God has done for us in the past. He's faithful. He wants you well, sweetheart. He is a good God who heals and answers prayer. He will see you through this."

I knew Dale was right. *God is good. And He loves me and wants me well. But I know I have to do my part.* He had promised me a way of escape. Now, I had to find it.

CHAPTER 7

Dressed Up with Nowhere to Go

*W*ednesday morning finally arrived, announced by a desert sunrise that created a postcard painting of purple and orange hues spreading over long-shadowed mountains. My internal angst stood in sharp contrast to the peaceful setting, but any fear of surgery was outweighed by the driving force to get cancer out of my body.

Dale and I held hands and prayed in the parking lot one last time before entering the all too familiar hospital. Once inside, I was speedily prepped for the operation. Since learning I had cancer, everything had led to this surgery. This was the big one—a radical mastectomy, removal of lymph nodes, and reconstruction. Dr. Anderson, my cancer surgeon, and Dr. Michaels, the reconstructive surgeon, stopped by to confirm our plan. The anesthesiologist followed, outlining what to expect.

Dale had been sitting beside me holding my hand since we arrived. Now it was time to say goodbye. With a tinge of fear tightening his face, Dale offered reassurance. "I'll keep praying for you, honey. My mom and our precious daughter, Kara, are in the waiting room. They're praying too. Don't forget, God is in control. He's going to lead us each step of the way. And we know His promises. He is already in the process of answering our prayers."

"I know, Dale. I'm counting on that." My heart was sure. My emotions . . . shaky.

"I love you, princess. I'll be waiting in recovery." As Dale stood to leave, I couldn't help but notice his eyes had welled up. I worried for him. He was trying to reassure me, but I knew he was struggling. I wanted to muster the strength to say something reassuring of my own.

All that came out was, "I love you too, Dale . . . so much."

He blew me a kiss and gave me a thumbs-up, then disappeared from view.

Alone. I was hit by a wall of panic. Then I remembered . . . *I'm not alone; I'm never alone. God is right here with me.*

Lord, I'm placing myself in Your care. I ask that You protect me through this surgery and guide the doctors' hands. I trust You, Father. I was ready.

The nurse headed my direction. "It's time, Paula. We're going to wheel you into surgery now." She was the same nurse I had when I had come in for the lumpectomy. We had spent several minutes just getting acquainted before that first surgery, and she had remembered me when I arrived this morning. I felt as though she really cared. Encouraging me with her smile, she and an orderly rolled my bed through the double doors of the OR, where we were immediately engulfed by a wall of frigid air. The warm blankets they draped over my body felt heavenly.

My bed was positioned in the center of the room and locked in place under glaring lights. Suddenly I felt a warm hand on each side of my head as the anesthesiologist, sitting above me, bent over my face and winked. I kept telling myself to breathe and everything would be okay. God was with me.

"Okay, Paula. I'm going to place this mask over your face, and I'd like you to start counting backward from a hundred. Can you do that for me?"

I nodded. "One hundred . . . ninety-nine . . . ninety-eight . . . ninety . . ." Blackness enveloped me.

"Paula, can you hear me? Paula. Paula. Wake up." *Who's trying to wake me up? The surgery just started.*

"Paula, you're in recovery. How are you feeling?" The nurse kept patting my hand as I forced my eyes open. My throat felt scratchy. Trying to gather my thoughts and remember what was happening took every ounce of focus.

"Can you hear me?" Her persistence seemed unnecessary.

"Yes, I can." My voice sounded raspy.

"Your surgery was aborted. I'm sorry."

I was sure I had misheard. "What? What happened?" My words slurred. "I don't understand. What do you mean?" *That doesn't make sense. Why would the surgery be aborted?*

Dr. Anderson arrived next to my bed and took over the explanation. "I'm sorry, Paula, but you are full of staph infection. We cannot proceed. We had to close you back up. We'll have to do the surgery after the infection clears. Do you understand me?"

"So the cancer is still in my body . . . growing? Are you kidding me?"

"It won't take that long to clear up the infection, and we'll reschedule you as soon as we can. Don't you worry—you're going to be okay." He patted my shoulder, trying to instill calm. "I'll check back with you in a few minutes."

But everyone was there to operate. Everything was ready. How could this have happened?

About that time, Dale showed up with widened eyes

of shock, having been summoned from the waiting room. I blurted out the news, hoping that by saying the words they might sink in. "I have a staph infection. They just closed me back up and postponed the surgery."

"I know, Paula." Dale rolled his eyes. "They told me. I'm so sorry." He spoke slowly, curbing his temper. "Believe me, I am not happy about this." His nostrils flared as he mumbled, "I wish I didn't know so much about hospitals."

"I can't believe this is happening. Cancer is still growing in my body and I feel helpless to do anything." Every negative emotion was jostling for position. *How can this be happening? How could God have allowed this?*

Dale's words bristled with irritation. "Apparently the first surgery caused the infection, Paula."

My problem had just been compounded with a dangerous, potentially lethal infection. Later, I would learn from other sources that for all intents and purposes, I had no working immune system whatsoever. My immune system was completely shot.

As if on cue, Dr. Anderson re-entered the room braced for questions. And Dale had the questions.

"Doctor, what's going on? How could this happen?" Dale's voice stung with unfriendliness. "Did we really have to abort this today? Her cancer is still growing—right? I mean no disrespect, but I'm upset." Dale was struggling to throttle back his emotions.

I knew Dale was revisiting his own experiences in the hospital—over a dozen surgeries he had endured following the airplane crash. He had shared his acquired distrust of the medical system with me after watching numerous friends die in hospitals because of what appeared to be incompetence. He knew all too well the risks involved in being in a hospital. The statistics of hospital-induced deaths caused by negligence and human error were staggering. And though he had been careful not to mention them prior to my surgery, I hadn't forgotten what he had shared throughout the years since his accident.

Dale was relentless in probing for information and had learned to question everything. I could see he was prepared to do it again.

Finally, struggling to calm himself, Dale went on. "Exactly when do you think we'll be able to make another attempt at surgery?"

"I know you're both frustrated," replied Dr. Anderson. "This is a rare occurrence, and there's nothing we can do at this point." Dale rolled his eyes again and looked away. Dr. Anderson nervously shifted his weight. "We have to treat the infection first—that's standard procedure. Once the infection has cleared, then, and only then, can we do the surgery."

The memories of what Dale had shared throughout the years marched through my mind. More people die each year from *preventable* medical errors in hospitals than from breast cancer and automobile accidents combined.

Thinking back, I remembered how devastated Dale was when his golf partner, Charley, a very dear friend, was admitted to the hospital for a simple, routine test. The nurse administered too much morphine. Within seconds, Dale's friend went into a coma. He was pronounced dead five days later.

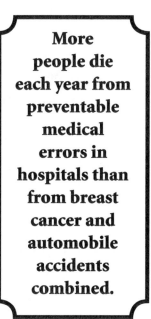

More people die each year from preventable medical errors in hospitals than from breast cancer and automobile accidents combined.

Then there was our next-door neighbor, Thomas, a retired airline pilot who had been taken to the hospital complaining of lower back pain. During the testing, he was given too much sedative and died.

The list grew to dozens of precious

people in Dale's life who had died needlessly because of human mistakes in hospitals.

Besides the personal examples of hospital error, there were the statistics Dale had shared with me. In an issue of the *Journal of the American Medical Association,* it was documented that over 225,000 deaths each year result from a doctor's activity, manner, or therapy. The study went on to state that by prescribing toxic drugs, performing unnecessary surgeries, or simply making a mistake, doctors are causing the deaths of hundreds of thousands of patients every year. This study reveals that annual deaths from such causes include the following: 12,000 because of unnecessary surgery; 80,000 from infections in hospitals; 7,000 from medication errors in hospitals; 106,000 from negative effects of drugs; and 20,000 because of other hospital errors. That makes America's healthcare-system-induced deaths the third leading cause of death in the U.S. after heart disease and cancer.[16]

That is a lot of people killed—in hospitals! And 80,000 from infections! The problem, it seemed to me, was that although most doctors may be responsible medical professionals, they are working in a broken system.

What mistake caused the infection I was dealing with? Was it a hospital error? *It doesn't matter now. I just want to know how much longer I have to live with this cancer growing in my body.*

"How long, doctor?" I asked. "When can we get to the cancer?"

"Probably about four weeks. I'll give you a prescription for some strong antibiotics that should knock this infection out. We'll reschedule as soon as you've finished taking them. How does that sound?" Dr. Anderson looked worried. I wasn't sure if it was because of the cancer spreading in my body—or if it was because he now knew that Dale, although a kind and gentle man on one hand, was not a pushover like so many patients.

Dr. Anderson wrote out the prescription and handed it to Dale as he finished talking to me. "I'll have my office give you a call with a new surgery date. You're going to be released to go home today. The nurse will be back in a few minutes to help you prepare to leave. And please fill that prescription in the pharmacy downstairs on your way out. You need to get started on the antibiotics immediately." Doc seemed anxious to leave. That was the first time I had seen him rattled.

As the doctor left, I turned to my husband. "Dale, please sit down. You're too upset."

"Are we supposed to just accept this? Who's running this place—the three stooges? How could this happen? Paula, staph infections that exist in the same location as a previous surgery are almost always caused by things being unsterile. We're in a hospital, for Pete's sake." Dale paced the floor, visibly agitated. Our lives were overflowing with challenges already, and someone had just thrown a hand grenade on top.

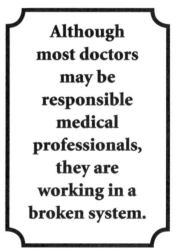

Although most doctors may be responsible medical professionals, they are working in a broken system.

Interrupted by the nurse's arrival, Dale headed to the pharmacy to get my prescription filled while I dressed and gathered my personal belongings.

Within an hour, we were on our way back home. This was not at all what I had imagined. I needed some alone time—just God and me. I had to figure out what was going on. Did He really promise me a way of escape . . . or had I completely messed up and misunderstood somehow? I thought God was guiding me, leading me, taking care of me. His promise had instilled hope for deliverance from this deadly disease. Why would He allow this delay in my healing? It didn't make sense.

If God isn't on my side . . . if He isn't answering my prayers . . . then I'm in serious trouble. A wave of fear rushed in like a tsunami—and I was drowning in terror. My fragile faith vanished.

I went into prayer-overdrive. *Where are You, God? How could You let this happen?*

CHAPTER 8

Body, Soul, and Spirit

⌒

"*P*aula, the car is loaded and ready to go. Do you need my help?"

"No, I can make it to the car, but can you get my Bible and purse?"

"No problem on the Bible, but you know I don't carry purses." Dale grinned as he scooped up both and headed to the car.

Dale and I were on our way to visit Jada in Riverside. She and I had stayed in touch through frequent phone conversations since meeting in the doctor's office and had formed a very special friendship. She knew I was struggling, and I hoped the trip would help get me out of my depression.

It had been almost two weeks since the staph infection was discovered and my surgery aborted. The setback was exceptionally hard to handle, and I was still reeling. Emotionally, I had gone down the drain. Nothing seemed to help. Dr. Anderson's words haunted me. "Your cancer is aggressive. You'll need radical surgery, full chemotherapy, and radiation treatments. And I believe if you don't do all these, you'll not be alive in three to six months." It had been almost a month—and I'd done nothing. Whatever traction I had acquired before surgery had vanished. Fear was back on the throne, jeering at me.

In addition to my melancholy, my body had taken on a life of its own. New symptoms were surfacing daily and driving me further underwater. Cancer was growing and spreading and becoming more obvious by the day. Fresh swelling under my left arm further empowered the kingdom of fear. *The cancer must have spread to my lymph nodes. It's getting worse.*

Just the day before, while taking a shower, I discovered a lump about the size of an almond on my forearm. My heart lurched. The lump was hard and didn't move when I rubbed it. Apparently it was attached to the bone. It just lay there under my skin, mocking me—and growing.

As if these symptoms weren't enough, a radiating pain had developed in my abdomen and hip. Walking even a short distance was painful and becoming increasingly difficult. My body was on a fast track toward self-destruction. New problems were setting up shop seemingly overnight. I felt as though I was stuck in a body controlled by something else—something alien.

My immune system was shot. That was abundantly clear. But until I was diagnosed with cancer, I had felt bulletproof. I thought I was healthier than almost anyone I knew. The years had been kind to me. Not an ounce overweight and fairly athletic, I enjoyed frequent outdoor activities. I was almost never sick and rarely visited the doctor. That made my physical challenges even more difficult to accept.

In my typical fashion, I rarely talked about my symptoms. Stirring up fear in those who loved me was something I tried to avoid. Fear is contagious and I had neither the resources nor stamina for their reactions and questions. Reducing my emotional footprint had become a top priority.

Lord, what are we doing? Where are You? Here I sit— waiting. And waiting. I need to do something to make things better. Now! But the doctor said all I can do is wait for the antibiotics. I feel like everything is falling apart. Have I done something to mess things up?

Wrestling with images of cancer cells spreading like wildfire compelled me to take a fresh look at what I knew about God and how He heals.

While driving west on Highway 10 toward Jada's house, I decided to revisit lessons Dale had learned while seeking healing after the airplane crash.

"Okay, Dale. Help me see how the principles you discovered relate to cancer and the threat I'm dealing with. I'm confused. And right now, I'm panicking. How did you deal with fear and anxiety?"

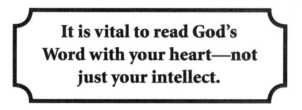

It is vital to read God's Word with your heart—not just your intellect.

"Paula, most everything I learned you already know, but let's review. I realized there were three vital parts I had to focus on— my body, soul, and spirit. First, my spiritual life. As you know, we are made in God's image so we are spiritual beings. The Bible describes our spirit and our heart as being the same. I diligently pursued the things of God. I learned about God and His desires for each of us. I also discovered what God responds to. I did this primarily through prayer and studying the Bible with an open mind *and* an open heart. Paula, it was vital for me to read God's Word with my heart, not just my intellect. The Word of God is

85

food for our spirit. By absorbing 'spirit food,' I grew faster and stronger in understanding God and His ways."

"Where did you read in the Bible, Dale? Just anywhere?"

"I focused most of my Bible study on the life of Jesus in the gospels. Since the Bible tells us that Jesus is the reflection of God and He did nothing except what God told Him to do, I figured I'd learn a lot about God's will by reading about the life of Jesus. Though I read other books of the Bible as well, it was primarily in the books of Matthew, Mark, Luke and John that it became clear that God's will was to heal me.

"While I was dealing with my spirit, I was also dealing with my soul. The soul is made up of the mind, the will, and the emotions. My soul was an equally important part to have functioning properly. God taught me how to keep my emotions in check by building faith in Him through His Word and by speaking and believing His promises. I call this 'heart-talk.' After all, I wanted His will, not mine. God's Word *is* His will. I learned to speak the promises of God every day, which changed how I felt and how I thought.

"Third, Paula, and just as important, I was dealing with my body. My brain had sustained enormous blunt trauma, which is what killed the other pilots. My body was broken and slashed in so many places it was overwhelming. I worked hard to exercise the injured areas, even exercising the muscles in my eyes, which had to overcome devastating damage so I could see again from my right eye. To get my memory back, I had to constantly challenge my mind—and that took years. And even while consigned to a wheelchair, I had to faithfully work out my body. My right side healed faster than my left so I would exercise the right side until the left side was able. The whole process took about seven years before I was relatively normal again.

"Paula, it's critical that you also deal with all three parts of your being. You'll be tending to your body, your soul, and your spirit. All three affect one another. Now you and I know a lot already about the spirit. We know the Bible and try to live by it. And you've done a great job in the area of your soul, at least until this last setback. But I know you'll bounce back. You usually speak the right way, you think the right way, and your positive can-do attitude makes you the type of person who doesn't wallow. But I think our greatest weakness right now is that we don't know about the body as it relates to cancer. We don't know exactly what causes this stinkin' disease, so obviously, we don't yet know the best ways to combat it. Overall, if you focus on a three-pronged approach—your body, your soul, and your spirit—then I firmly believe you will succeed at beating this menacing threat of cancer."

"Okay, Dale, I get it—body, soul, and spirit. Those three parts make up the complete me, and they are interconnected so each affects the others. That makes complete sense. Wasn't your ankle one of your biggest answers to prayer? Did that healing involve your body, soul, and spirit?"

"Oh, yes. Absolutely. First, the doctor told me I'd never walk again. Months later he believed I might be able to eventually put weight on my foot if I had a third specialized surgery. The good news was, if successful, I would walk again. The bad news was that I'd have no ankle joint and would walk with a severe limp. I would be crippled for life."

"The surgery would have put an end to your baseball scholarship, not to mention your dream of being an airline pilot."

"That's right, Paula, but the fact that I was alive was a miracle. And believe me, I was grateful. I knew God had spared my life. Just as the Bible promised, I drew near to Him and He drew near to me. God became very real and personal."

"But, Dale, what about healing? Tell me about God's will for my healing of cancer. What did you learn that can help me now?"

Dale grabbed my hand. "Oh, Paula, of course I'm going to help in every way I can. That's what I'm here to do, sweetheart. Look, I learned through studying the Bible that it was God's will for me to be healed. Isaiah prophesied, 'But He was wounded for our transgressions, He was bruised for our iniquities; the chastisement for our peace was upon Him and by His stripes we are healed.' And 1 Peter 2:24 says, '. . . by whose stripes you *were* healed.' The verb there, in the original, is past tense. Eventually I realized that healing from God was *already* mine through what Jesus accomplished on the cross. It was a done deal. My healing—just like my salvation—had been paid for already by the blood of Jesus. By spending so much time in prayer and in God's Word, I felt like God's Spirit was with me everywhere I went, helping me think the way I should and helping me understand His ways.

"And, Paula, when I studied the life of Jesus, I noticed that He healed every person who came to Him. He turned no one down. He never said no to anyone who came to Him with an open heart." Dale paused and lifted his index finger. "There's one exception. When Jesus was in Nazareth, the Bible said He could not do many miracles there because of their unbelief. Unbelief keeps us from receiving God's best. Faith in God's Word is what overcomes unbelief."

> **Healing from God is already yours through what Jesus accomplished on the cross.**

"That's wonderful, and I already believe that, Dale. But what about my next surgery? It's coming up soon, and I have to decide what to do about chemo and radiation. How did you decide which path to take—surgery or no surgery?"

"I needed and wanted God's direction." Dale stopped speaking while he transitioned our car onto the 60 freeway while passing through the city of Beaumont. Taking advantage of the interlude in our conversation, I scanned the people in the cars around us. Everyone was headed somewhere. So many people—such busy lives. *Do any of them have cancer?*

Once established on our new heading, Dale resumed speaking. "I knew the Bible would guide me, so I prayed. I asked God to reveal His will for me. Then I'd read my Bible with an open heart. One particular time I was reading the gospel of Matthew, and a scripture jumped off the page at me. Just like what happened to you with your promise from God about finding your way of escape. That's exactly how it happened to me. Do you remember Matthew, chapter seven, verses seven and eight?"

"Absolutely. 'Ask, and it will be given to you; seek, and you will find; knock, and it will be opened to you. For everyone who asks receives, and he who seeks finds, and to him who knocks it will be opened.' I remember you saying that you almost couldn't breathe when you read that."

Dale choked up and wiped a few tears from his eyes. "Yes, that's the verse. It still impacts me today. Reading it was as exciting as if I had found buried treasure. I believed in my heart I had found my answer: 'Don't have the third surgery but ask God for complete healing.' So I prayed and believed God would answer my prayers and heal my ankle—and that I'd be able to walk again.

"When I made public the decision that I wasn't going to have the surgery, those close to me thought I was crazy. Some tried to change my mind. I don't need to remind you that my ankle was completely destroyed in the crash. But I felt I had heard from God. Unfortunately, the bone was dying more every day. Finally, I had waited too long. Remember, Paula, I wasn't dealing with life and death like you are. My issues were physical and emotional but not life threatening."

"I know, Dale, but still it helps to review your story. Keep going. This is encouraging."

"Well, honey, over time my faith developed. I finally had confidence that I knew what God's will was for me. After rejecting the third surgery, I kept returning to the doctor for X-rays, expecting to hear the doctor say my ankle was healed. It didn't happen that way. At every appointment, the X-rays showed the ankle getting worse. Finally, the bone was dead." Dale punctuated the statement by lifting his leg and slapping his left ankle. "Once the bone died, surgery was no longer an option. I felt blindsided. That's when faith drained out of me and fear flooded in. I started questioning everything. Had I made a mistake? Did I misunderstand? Where was God?"

> **God's promises are more credible than your physical symptoms.**

"That's how I'm feeling, Dale. So you were afraid you'd be crippled the rest of your life? I mean totally crippled because by then nothing more could be done." I relentlessly probed for more information. "So how did you deal with your fears? That's my biggest problem since the staph infection and the aborted surgery. I'm becoming frantic. And now there's this lump on my arm and pain in my abdomen. Talk about fear—the cancer is obviously spreading. And I can't do any treatments at all for now except take antibiotics, which does *nothing* for the cancer."

"I have to admit, Paula, your symptoms are overwhelming to me too. I'm sorry to admit it, but your cancer is the biggest challenge I've ever faced." I could tell from his voice, Dale was as frightened as I was about our predicament. He continued, "But even in the midst of this, we have to remember God's promises are more credible than your physical symptoms. Believe me, I know how fear can take over. It's that sick feeling in your stomach when you think you've made a life-altering mistake and it's too late to change it. You know, Paula, I couldn't sleep for days after my anklebone died. The fear was almost incapacitating. Yet I was only dealing with the ability to walk again, not life and death."

"Well, still, the principles are what I'm looking for, Dale. The fear you described is exactly how I feel. My stomach tightens and I get these knots in my gut. I feel hot and panicky . . . like i'm doomed. And it seems like there's nothing I can do to change the outcome. I'm afraid of making the biggest mistake of my life. Afraid I'll make a fatal miscalculation as we get into the treatments. What if I choose to have chemo and it's the wrong choice? Or what if I don't do the mastectomy and the cancer gets worse? I need confidence in whatever decision I make. Right now, I'm paralyzed. How did you get past the point of debilitating fear?"

"Gosh, Paula, I kept reading the Bible. But I did more than read. I studied it, and I found promises about healing and who God is. As I learned about His will for me, I spoke those promises of God aloud. Since the Bible says, 'Faith comes by hearing and hearing by the word of God,'[17] I would also play Bible tapes every night—all night long. As you know, I've continued doing that ever since the crash. Every time I heard myself speaking words rooted in God's Word, my faith would grow and the fear would diminish. It's a lot like turning on a light in a dark room. The light forces out the darkness just as faith chases out the fear. I did that for weeks and weeks. It was a real battle, Paula.

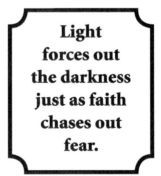

Light forces out the darkness just as faith chases out fear.

"Then one day I went back to the doctor for my usual X-ray. This time the doctor was shocked by what he saw. My dead anklebone had new life in it! The blood had started circulating again. The bone was healing. It took a few years, but eventually the blood circulation was complete—I was able to walk again.

As you know, the most difficult times of life can become the best times of life if we let God direct them. That's what I've experienced. And that can happen for you too, sweetheart."

"I know that's true. Thanks for the encouragement. It helps to hear it again—and again. God miraculously healed your ankle, but everything else just took a lot of hard work."

"That's a fact, Paula. It was one of the most difficult and challenging times of my life."

Just then we pulled off the freeway, only a few blocks from the address Jada had given us.

"Dale, I need more time and focus to sort things out. Do you think we could somehow get away for a few days?"

Trying to lighten the mood, Dale pushed back his baseball cap and peered at me, his expression serious. I was preparing to hear another pearl of inspiration and wisdom that would solve my problem when he uttered, "Well, Paula, you've got to ask yourself one question."

"Okay. What's that?"

Dale smirked, lowered his voice, and in his best Dirty Harry impersonation said, "Do you feel lucky?"

"Oh, my gosh!" I shook my head in disbelief. "I thought you were serious."

Dale grinned broadly. Now lowering his sunglasses, he stared at me for a second. "Well, do ya . . . punk?"

Punching his shoulder, all I could do was chuckle as I shook my head. Dale howled in such rollicking laughter, he had trouble staying in his lane. I wondered if I could be arrested for spousal abuse because of all the bruising I caused by punching him on his arm and leg and elbowing him in his side. *I need to be careful.* I smiled. *He could report me.*

We chatted about lighter things until pulling up at Jada's daughter's house, where Jada had been living since starting the second round of chemo. Jada and I had become close. Even though we were struggling with a deadly disease, we both believed God would heal us. Several times each week, we shared our faith and prayed together on the phone. When one of us was down, the other was the encourager. As our relationship grew, it became apparent Jada needed me as much as I needed her.

As I exited the car, the front door of the house flew open and Jada charged in our direction. We met halfway and collided in a long hug, rocking each other back and forth in a warm embrace.

On the outside, Jada and I couldn't have looked more different. She was short and stocky, a black woman from the Deep South. I was tall and slim with long blond hair and blue eyes, originally from Idaho. Jada was several years my senior and spoke with an attractive southern drawl. But as different as we looked on the outside, we felt like sisters. We acted like sisters—because that's exactly what we were. You see, Jada and I shared the unique bond of love and unity as members of the family of God. Spiritually speaking, we *were* sisters.

The bond between Jada and me had grown stronger as we shared our faith and prayed together several times on the phone. Having another Christian woman who was dealing with cancer, one I could talk to, had been a real help.

Raised in a small town near Memphis, Jada and her husband had attended the same Baptist Church for twenty-two years. They had moved to southern California five years earlier because of her husband's job transfer. Sadly, he had since passed away.

Jada was also believing that God would heal her. She had a good support group at her church and participated as often as her health would allow.

After a few precious hours of visiting with Jada and her daughter, it was time to head for home. Dale grabbed our hands and led us in prayer, asking God for guidance and His healing touch on our bodies.

As we said our goodbyes, I leaned over and hugged Jada again for the longest time. I closed my eyes, feeling her hair brush my neck as tears trickled down her cheek, dropping on my shoulder.

Our endearing embrace ended as she stepped back and clasped my hands. "With God's help, we'll get through this, sister. We're gonna beat this darn cancer."

"We will, Jada, we will." Tears filled my eyes. Jada and I both knew—more than most—every moment was precious, and life was uncertain at best. "Thank you for inviting us over. It was just what I needed."

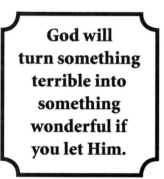

God will turn something terrible into something wonderful if you let Him.

Jada flashed her thousand-watt smile, then turned and grabbed a small bag sitting on the counter. "Here's a little somethin' for the road."

We hadn't driven a block before Dale asked, "What's that I smell? It smells like cookies."

I opened the bag to find six freshly baked chocolate chip cookies. "Oh, that Jada. She is such a sweetheart."

"No kidding, Paula. The two of you have an amazing bond. I'm so glad you found each other."

"I am too, Dale. She is a real gift from God. Jada will be a friend for life."

Back on the freeway, after sampling a couple of cookies, Dale recalled our earlier conversation and asked if I wanted to pick it up where we had left off. I did.

"Dale, we were talking before about your fears after the airplane crash. Seriously, honey. What did you do about them? I'm scared and I don't know how to get past the fear."

"Learning how to fight fear with faith was one of the keys to my success. And, Paula, faith is also the key to your battle with cancer. The principles are the same, and God doesn't change.

You *will* beat cancer. I know it *is* God's will for you to be well—to have victory over this darn disease. First, honey, you'll need to fight a colossal battle with your faith. It almost always takes a fight of faith to receive God's will in this world."

"Can I ask you another question, Dale? This might be a tough one. What do you say to those who think God caused the crash?"

"Oh, I don't believe God caused the airplane to crash—but He did allow it. God didn't stop it from happening, yet He could have. Just like He didn't stop you from getting cancer. Paula, I don't believe for a second that God caused cancer in your body. That is not like God. Something else has caused this cancer, yet God has allowed it. Soon we're going to learn why. Then we're going to find out what we can do about it. That's just one of the wonderful things about God. He will turn something terrible into something wonderful if we let Him."

"Yes, Dale, but I need to make sure my perspective is accurate and my battle plan is scripturally sound. You eventually won your battle, but what if I lose mine? What if I die this year or the next? Gosh, what if I die in the next few months?" Verbalizing my deepest fears proved more stressful than I had imagined. I stared out the window, silently watching the landscape go by. Death was difficult to discuss.

Finally, Dale interrupted the silence. "Well, sweetheart, I sure don't like talking about that. But I don't want to bury my head in the sand either. And I'm not encouraging you to deny the seriousness of the facts. But we shouldn't pray and believe one way and then speak the opposite. That never produces good results. This one time, okay, let's discuss you losing your battle with cancer and dying like many friends and family we have

> **Praying and believing one way and speaking the opposite never produces good results.**

known. But this should be the only time we do this, Paula. The *only* time."

Dale and I spent the rest of the drive home discussing the possibility of my life ending if I lost my battle with cancer. Through many tears, I shared the biggest regrets I would have. Fear of death was not among them. It was the fear of not being here for our children and for Dale. Missing those all-important life events like weddings and grandchildren, not celebrating the victories and special experiences or being there to offer support and share the tears of painful circumstances that were sure to invade the lives of those I loved. My grandparents and parents were supposed to die before me. Leaving behind all the precious people in my life would be my greatest regret. I was a wife, mother, daughter, sister, and friend. I couldn't imagine not being there as all those lives continued on. It seemed so wrong. So unfair. I yearned to keep living. There was still so much to live for.

Our conversation continued as I poured out all my thoughts, my fears, my regrets. We both cried and even laughed occasionally. I shared where I wanted to be buried, the dress I wanted to wear in my coffin, what songs were important at my funeral service, and which picture to use. So many details, but all important ones if I was going to die. Surprisingly, it actually felt good to put into words all the thoughts that had been tormenting me for weeks. Death is so much a part of life—always there, motivating us in ways we don't consciously consider. Death is inevitable. *True, but not yet. It's way too soon.* As we neared home, I had said all I needed to say. The window of discussion was now closing—and I would never try to open that window again.

Not a word was spoken the rest of the trip and by the time we pulled into the garage, Dale and I were spent. We sat in silence, neither of us ready to leave our solemn cocoon.

Dale placed a soft hand on my knee, "Keep pressing in,

Paula. Remember the scripture says, 'Draw near to God, and He will draw near to you.'[18] From personal experience, I can promise that if you keep pursuing God, not just what He can do for you but God Himself, you won't be disappointed. You'll find what you're looking for."

"This has helped a lot, Dale. I don't have time to lose. I have to dig into His Word, to fight fear with faith, to find His answers—His timing. Believing God wants me well is the cornerstone of whatever plan I choose to follow. I know I don't have the power to fix this. But God does."

I was dueling with death. And this was a fight I *had* to win.

> **Believing God wants you well is the cornerstone of whatever plan you choose to follow.**

CHAPTER 9

Heading for the Hills

⤳

*S*ummer had arrived in full force. Though the desert heat was already wearing on me, it was no match for the incessant harassment of the telephone. It wouldn't stop ringing and I wanted to scream!

It's not that I didn't appreciate the care and concern people were showing. But, wow, the repeated questions—the same ones over and over: "How are you doing?" "What are you going to do?" *How am I doing? I am confused and frustrated and afraid. And I have no idea what I'm going to do!*

It seemed like everyone in my life knew I had cancer. Bad news *does* travel fast. Not only did they ask what I was going to do—they told me what they thought I *should* do. Advice came from every direction.

I had no idea cancer had touched so many lives. Almost everyone I spoke with knew someone with cancer. Their uncle or cousin or best friend had cancer and treated it this way or that. There was no shortage of recommendations.

"Good grief, Dale," I finally said, "I don't think I can handle one more call. I mean, I know their intentions are all good. I know they're trying to show they care. But the constant bombardment is more than I can handle. What can I do? I don't want to offend anyone by not taking their call, but I can't keep going like this. I have no time to think, no time to process. I need quiet. I need time alone with God to figure out how He is leading me."

"I understand, honey. Let's turn down the volume. Just answer the calls you want and let the others go to voicemail. Let them all go to voicemail, as far as I'm concerned. We'll deal with them later."

"Oh, good. I'm so tired and overwhelmed."

"Don't worry, Paula. I'll change the phone message. The only time you should use a telephone is if *you* want to call someone." I nodded in relief. "You're on overload right now, and that's understandable. Hey, here's an idea. What do you say we pack our bags and get out of Dodge? Forget everything else. Nothing is more important than you having some peace and a place to sort things out. On our trip to Jada's, that's what you told me you needed. Are you with me on this?"

"Dale, I'm supposed to show up at work tomorrow. And you have responsibilities with the church. How do we just pack up and drive away?"

"We just do it. Paula, nothing is more important than dealing with your cancer. Why don't you make a call to your employer and ask for a leave of absence. If that doesn't work, I suggest you quit. And I'll ask Rick to preach for me this week, and for as many weeks as we need. Everything else can wait."

"Really? Are you serious?"

"Oh, I'm *very* serious. You're dealing with a deadly disease. There is no way you're going to be able to work *and* fight this battle at the same time. Me neither, for that matter. I can't do all the research your situation requires and work full time too. Paula, the cancer already appears to have spread significantly.

This is life and death. Jobs, money—those things aren't that important in light of what you're dealing with."

"That's true. And I need some quality time away—not just a quick weekend. But where will we go?"

Dale smiled. "I've been planning a surprise for a while, Paula. Mike and Joanie offered us their cabin, and I've already made the arrangements. We're all set. Let's take the dog and whatever essentials we need and get out of town. What do you think?"

"That sounds wonderful. It's exactly what I need. To be somewhere alone with God and hear what He has to say." Relief swept over me. This was the right step.

Dale and I made a few phone calls and cleared our calendars for the immediate future. As it would turn out, I'd never go back to my job. And Dale would never go back to pastor the church he and I had planted.

Dr. Anderson had me on a month-long regime of strong antibiotics to clear the infection. Unless I found a better plan soon, I would go under the knife again for the radical mastectomy, immediately followed by full-scale chemo and radiation treatments. Decisions would be required from me within days. There was no time to lose.

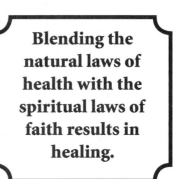

Blending the natural laws of health with the spiritual laws of faith results in healing.

"Dale, this is the perfect time to get more books for the research we're doing on cancer and treatment options. Let's pick some up and take them with us to the mountains. That's the perfect place to focus, don't you think?"

"Bingo, Paula. That's exactly what we should do. And didn't you say your mom is sending you a package? What's that about?"

"It's the story of a medical doctor, a woman who was cured

of breast cancer. It wasn't a miraculous healing, but she did what you did after the airplane crash—blending natural laws of health with spiritual laws of faith in God. She was cured of advanced stage breast cancer without any conventional treatment whatsoever."

Dale perked up. "That sounds promising. What did she do, exactly?"

"I don't know, but Mom said I need to review her materials. This woman had a huge tumor. Dale, it was the size of my fist. She turned to God for the first time in her life and somehow got well without doing any surgery and without any chemo or radiation. Mom said she's overnighting her material to us. It would be terrific if it arrives before we leave."

"You're right, but I don't think we should delay our trip. We'll have more than enough research materials without that. You know, Paula, where the Bible says, 'My people are destroyed for lack of knowledge'?[19] Remember that verse?"

"Of course."

"Well, I bring it up now for one reason—this will *not* be you. We're going to learn everything we need to learn to beat cancer. Between the information we'll learn and the wisdom God provides, we will find your way of escape, sweetheart. I guarantee it."

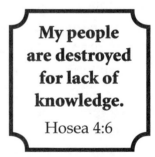

My people are destroyed for lack of knowledge.

Hosea 4:6

"That sounds perfect to me, Dale. I can be ready to leave in thirty minutes."

Our first stop was the library. Though Dale had previously checked out several books, we searched for anything else that looked promising. There were dozens of books and an abundance of medical journals. Never had I imagined so much had been written about cancer or realized the enormous place it held in our society.

We spent a couple of hours inside the library, each of

us scurrying in different directions. We read, scanned, and evaluated all the resources available—an amazing amount of information. When we finally checked out, we were both carrying two armloads of books and journals.

Dale leaned over and whispered in jest, "We're going to need a bigger boat."

I smiled. *How are we going to get through all this material?*

"What about the bookstore, Paula? Shouldn't we take a look there before we leave town? We need all the resources we can get."

Dale didn't know how to face a challenge halfway. He was always scrupulously thorough. *Why can't I be the same way?*

At the bookstore, I was amazed to find a multitude of books on cancer we had not found in the library. Dale and I pulled book after book from the shelves. We didn't have much money to spend, but nothing was more important than getting the information we needed. After skimming through the mountain of books, we narrowed it down to eight that we just *had* to have.

Back in the car, I realized I'd forgotten something important at the house. Usually reluctant to backtrack, Dale agreed to return, determined to help me with whatever I needed. When we pulled up at the house, we looked at each other and smiled. Neither of us felt the need to comment as we watched the FedEx driver walking back to his truck. He'd left a package at the door—a box from Mom with the materials she had promised.

The higher we climbed the mountain roads, the more I sensed the stress fading. *I really need this time.* I hadn't realized how much pressure I was dealing with until the tension started peeling away.

Just before the road turned deeper into the hills, Dale pulled off at a desert overlook, a large space carved out of the mountainside where cars pulled over to view the entire valley below. Dale took Wicket, our little Lhasa apso, out for a brief walk. I smiled to myself remembering how our children had chosen the dog and his name. At ages seven and five they had fallen in love with Wicket, the leader of the Ewoks in one of the *Star Wars* movies. I had to admit, our dog looked *exactly* like an Ewok.

That was fourteen years earlier. I shook my head, marveling at how quickly time had flown by. Sitting in the car gazing out over the desert community, my eyes fell on the well-known hospital where I had already endured two surgeries. I stared down at the familiar neighborhood where we lived. I could see the avenue where we shopped for wigs and the area where our church was situated. My thoughts turned to the many people I had met since being diagnosed with cancer: my doctors, the oncologist, the nurses, and so many others. I had made new friends like Jada and the four others in the "cancer club." I reflected on the people in our church, our neighbors, our family, our friends, and, of course, Eric and Kara, our two wonderful children.

So much had already happened in the valley below. I was looking over the backdrop where my life's drama would play itself out during the next few months. A lot was going to change—that much I knew.

And with these thoughts came two haunting questions. *Will I find my way of escape? Or will I be dead by Christmas?*

CHAPTER 10

Mountain Madness

⮑

*R*esting high in the San Jacinto Mountains, Idyllwild is nestled among tall pines, sweet-smelling cedars, and legendary rocks. With a population of only 3,800, it has the quintessential small town atmosphere. The locale is a favorite for weekend rock climbers and hikers, but is best known as a haven for artists, boasting several art camps and schools. This mountain oasis high above the desert was the ideal place for the research and focus Dale and I needed.

Escaping the traffic and noisy city life, and of course the darn telephone, was giving me much needed peace. Tucked among the pines and hugging massive boulders, the rustic log cabin on the outskirts of town would become our ground zero.

It was a simple cabin, wrapped by an oversized covered porch that held several wooden chairs and a generous stack of firewood. A gray stone chimney pierced the steep green metal roof, further blending the cabin into the rugged landscape. The setting resembled a scene in a Thomas Kinkade painting, just waiting for the lights to go on.

After exploring the homey interior, decorated with worn

but comfortable furnishings, we stood on the back porch silently surveying the rocky canyon below. Dale put his arm around my waist and teased in a subdued voice, "Paula, I have a feeling we're not in Kansas anymore."

After Dale unloaded our belongings from the car and I got us settled in, we were ready for the task at hand—uncovering the mysteries of cancer. I stared at the huge pile of books on the kitchen table. *There must be more than forty books here. How are we supposed to get through all of them in a few days?* Once again, the challenge ahead seemed daunting.

Dale could see the distress on my face. "Don't worry, Paula. We'll figure it out. Let's just take one step at a time."

The task was beyond my natural ability. "Dale, can we pray about this?"

Dale faced me and grasped my hands. "Dear God. Paula and I ask for Your help as we search for her way of escape. Thank You for Your Word. Thank You for Your promises. Guide us through this mountain of information. Help us learn what You want us to learn. We give You authority over this process and our time together. And please continue Your healing touch in Paula's body. Give her peace that passes understanding. Thank You, dear Lord. Amen."

"Thanks honey. That ought to do it." I crossed the kitchen floor to open the refrigerator door. Empty. "Dale, we're going to need lots of energy to tackle this project."

"Oh, that's a fact. But we should dive right in. There's a lot of work to do."

"But we just got here. We haven't even had lunch. Surely, you're not serious."

"Oh, Paula, I *am* serious." Dale paused and looked me straight in the eye as I stared back in disbelief. Then he grinned. "And don't call me Shirley."

I couldn't help but laugh.

Dale grabbed the keys and said, "Let's go get lunch."

TWO DAYS LATER

After reading, searching, and devouring our respective stacks of journals, medical literature, and books of all sizes, we were both on information overload. I could only hope our questions would be answered and our confusion would be replaced with understanding.

A couple of days earlier, Dale and I had divided the books into two equal piles and had disappeared into separate rooms to begin our cancer education. Sequestered in the master bedroom and surrounded by books, I was engrossed in my quest for knowledge when Dale stepped through the door, looking as if he'd seen a ghost. "Paula, I can't read any more right now. I've got to talk. I can hardly believe what I've been learning—but sadly, I believe it."

"Believe what, Dale? What are you talking about?" I closed my book and gave him my full attention.

"Paula, I have read the first three chapters of twelve books. That's what I've been doing since we got here. I've studied the introductions, the prologues, the forewords—everything. And even with reading only the first three chapters of each book, I have discovered some shocking truths."

"Are you sure it's the truth?"

"Oh yeah! It's the truth all right. And as disheartening as it is, it's also a relief because now everything I know about cancer is making sense. As you know, that's what happens when one discovers the truth. Everything starts lining up."

"Well, what have you learned, Dale? Explain it to me."

"I'm not talking about facts, Paula. Facts are one thing—truth is another. With truth, there are no more mixed signals. Usually, truth is so hard to swallow that most people aren't open to it—not if they already believe something else. And then if they *do* hear the truth, they often go into denial or get angry—even hostile."

"I know, Dale. The truth can sometimes be hard to hear, especially if it contradicts what someone has come to believe. So, Dale—what have you learned?"

Dale began pacing back and forth across the room. 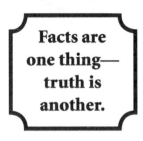 "Without full-scale treatments, you've been given a death sentence. Your cancer is advanced—and aggressive. But what I've learned tells me you are not going to be able to trust anyone. No one except God, that is. Paula, I'm shocked. I'm stunned, frustrated, and angry."

> Facts are one thing—truth is another.

"Wow, Dale! But you should know that I'm discovering some amazing things too—things that are knocking the wind out of me."

"Gosh, Paula, I am not surprised. Okay, who first? You or me?"

"Go ahead, Dale. Tell me why you're so upset."

"Well, first of all, let me say I've been studying for two long days, and it's taken everything in me not to share these things with you sooner. But I wanted to be absolutely certain I was discovering the truth. Now I *am* sure. Paula, if cancer is diagnosed early, and the right treatments are chosen, then finding a permanent cure is fairly easy. I'm talking permanent—not that five year mumbo-jumbo definition of cure. I know this sounds almost unbelievable, but honey, I'm now certain that this information is true. But here's the kicker. The way to treat cancer successfully is the opposite of everything I've heard my entire life."

"Oh my gosh, Dale. Really?"

"Yes. And based on what I've been learning, I believe God is answering our prayers. We are finding glimpses of the truth. On one hand, I'm thrilled. But on the other hand, this is gut-wrenching torture. There's nothing that gets me more riled up than knowing I've been lied to."

"As tough as this is, Dale, I want to know the truth. I don't want to bury my head just because it's difficult or new. If we don't have the truth to start with, how can we possibly make right choices?"

"As I mentioned a minute ago, Paula, a few types of cancer are so precarious that a person has to make perfect choices for treatment from the very beginning. The initial treatment has to be a bull's-eye right out of the gate because you don't get a second chance."

My heart started racing. "Is breast cancer one of those?" I held my breath.

"No, sweetheart. I'm glad to say breast cancer is not. Pancreatic cancer *is* one of those, and there are several others."

Uh-oh. Where is the pancreas? In the abdomen? Is that why I'm hurting there? I pushed the thought away so I could focus on what Dale was saying.

"Paula, all types of cancer are treatable and reversible. However . . ." Dale lifted his hand and paused, "some cancers are so serious, you don't get a second chance. But your odds improve dramatically by doing the 'right thing' the first time."

"Tell me more about successful cancer treatments being the opposite of everything you've ever heard or learned before. What does that mean?"

Dale finally stopped pacing and plopped into a chair, crossing his legs. "Well, we've talked a little about what cancer is, but I'm learning a lot more now. Remember, cancer cells are described more or less as undifferentiated cells. They multiply without uniformity. Unlike a healthy cell, a cancer cell has no useful function in the body. For example, cancer cells can't form muscle tissue. A cancer cell can't be part of the heart or become a useful part of any of the body's organs. In other words, cancer cells can't and don't do anything constructive.

They just sit there multiplying and robbing healthy cells of nutrients."

"Dale, that's what I'm learning too. When our immune system gets weak, the abnormal cells multiply faster than our immune system can destroy them. Everyone has cancer cells in their body all the time, but if we don't have enough white blood cells to kill off the cancer cells and keep them in check, a tumor will eventually form. And a tumor is nothing more than a grouping of cancer cells that multiply until the mass becomes large enough to detect. A tumor is just a *symptom* of cancer."

"Exactly, Paula. Tumors aren't cancer. Tumors are the *symptoms* of cancer." We looked at each other in astonishment.

I shook my head. "I've always thought that cancer was the tumor . . . but it's not."

Dale continued. "Cancer is the result of a broken immune system that allows cancer cells to duplicate and spread unchecked."

"Here's another thing, Paula. Cancer cells are only a small part of tumor tissue. Isn't that weird? Tumors are composed primarily of healthy cells."

> **Cancer is the result of a broken immune system that allows cancer cells to duplicate and spread unchecked.**

"I always assumed tumors *were* the cancer and they were made up of only cancer cells."

"Not true. Because most of the cells in a tumor are healthy, there generally aren't enough cancer cells inside a tumor to kill a person. No one ever dies of cancer cells inside a breast or inside a prostate gland, for example. Apparently some tumors have grown to well over one hundred pounds yet didn't kill the patient.

"It's not the tumor that kills, Paula. The spreading of cancer cells does. When cancer cells spread and multiply in large amounts, they can literally suck the life from the patient. They do this two ways—by taking vital nutrients out of healthy cells and then creating and releasing toxins into the body. So for cancer to kill a person, the cancer cells have to spread well beyond the tumor itself. Are you ready for more shocking news?"

"Sure. What's that?"

Dale stood, shook his head back and forth, and began pacing the floor again. "Oncology. Remember what we learned about the word *oncologist?*"

"Yeah, it means a doctor trained in the study and treatment of tumors. Right?"

"Right. So get this. The oncologist treats tumors. Hello-o-o? Is anybody listening? Paula! What's wrong with that picture?" Dale's nostrils flared open and closed like bellows. Everything in his body language screamed frustration.

"Oh my word." My fingers covered my mouth as I whispered. "The tumor isn't really the problem, is it?"

"Bull's-eye. That's right! They're not treating cancer—they are treating *symptoms.* Conventional medicine is not treating the cancer itself. The industry is treating the symptoms of cancer . . . not the root cause. No one will ever cure cancer by treating only symptoms. No way. This is sickening."

Can that be right? Chemo won't treat my cancer? My heart was pounding. "Dale, are you telling me if I have the chemotherapy my doctors have prescribed, it won't deal with my cancer?"

"That's exactly what I'm saying. Not only that, Paula, but the chemotherapy is harmful in two ways. First, it does *not* treat your cancer. Second, at the least, it greatly weakens your God-given immune system. Sometimes it even destroys it. Do you remember Carrie Walker?"

"Refresh my memory."

"Carrie had taken her mom to a chemotherapy treatment and afterward she was so sick she passed out in the car. She was pronounced dead on arrival at the hospital minutes later. The report showed she died of cancer, but Carrie believes she actually died from the chemotherapy drugs. Remember that?"

"Yes, now I do. That sounds like the story of Jada's cousin who died in the chemotherapy chair. Patients apparently get so weak and sick from the chemo that it's too much for their bodies to handle."

"Paula, this is happening all the time. Not everyone dies of chemotherapy treatments, but everyone is adversely affected. Everyone. There are *no* exceptions."

"That is so sad. As if cancer isn't bad enough, people have to worry about the treatments for cancer too. Incredible."

"Oh, Paula, it's more than sad. This is sickening." Dale threw up his hands. "I'm upset about it. And that's not all—there's still a lot more to share. Listen to what G. Edward Griffin says in his book *World Without Cancer.* 'If cancer patients undergoing these FDA-approved therapies were to read the actual laboratory reports, they would recoil in horror. They show neither safety nor effectiveness and, in fact, they are not intended to do so.'[20] Can you believe that?"

> **Chemotherapy can only slow down and shrink the cancer tumor. Meanwhile, it devastates the patient's immune system, making the cancer problem worse at the root level.**

"No wonder people are dying from chemotherapy treatments. Dale, I need to hear everything you're learning."

"Okay. And this still shocks me. I've found more confirmation that a person who takes enough chemo to kill all the cancer cells in their body will die from the toxicity of the chemo well before the cancer cells are destroyed? And chemotherapy doesn't *stop* cancer from spreading. In reality, many people die of the treatment long before the cancer kills them. Chemotherapy can only slow down and shrink the cancer tumor. Meanwhile, it devastates the patient's immune system, making the cancer problem worse at the root level. A weak immune system is what allows the cancer to grow out of control in the first place. Chemo is so toxic that I can't find *one* good reason to use it. Not even one. Not if we're trying to cure you of cancer."

"Good grief. Then why are all my doctors telling me to do it?"

"Partly because chemotherapy can put cancer into remission. Unfortunately, many cancer patients don't live long enough to go into remission. Then others go into remission several times. Tragically, remission is the goal for many in the medical industry, and patients are conditioned to be satisfied with that. But remission? Honey, I love you. And I need you. Why should we ask God for remission? I believe it's His will for you to be *cured* of cancer. It's not just my will I'm talking about here. I know in my heart that this is the will of God, Paula. It is God's best that you live a healthy, vibrant, long life on this earth."

I could feel the blood running out of my face as all this new information was sinking in. At the same time, I was wound up with tension.

"Paula, this must be so exhausting for you. Would you like to rest for a while?"

"No thanks, Dale. I'm too keyed up. I feel like I've had an adrenaline rush." I squeezed the arms of the chair. "I'm out of time. We have to figure this out and find God's answer for me. Go ahead—tell me what else you learned."

"Well, okay, let's talk about surgery and radiation. Surgery doesn't stop the cancer that has already spread. Often the cancer has spread beyond what a surgeon can cut out—that's exactly what happened to you. And surgery doesn't cure cancer in any way. At best, it simply removes a symptom."

"What about radiation? I remember you told me it could damage the healthy cells, so it doesn't sound like a good answer either."

"You're right, Paula. Radiation does *not* attack the root of the cancer. Plus it's damaging and counterproductive. Radiation is like shooting cancer cells with a bullet—and bullets just do more damage." Dale's voice raised two decibels. "And get this! Radiation therapy can actually *cause* cancer. How's that for treatment?"

"Unbelievable."

"No kidding. Here we are, asking God for a permanent cure, yet the only thing your doctors are trying to do is shrink the tumors. What are they doing for the cancer? It's maddening. We're expecting the doctors to cure you of cancer by not treating your cancer? Goodness gracious. Shrinking the tumor can't be the goal. What's going on here?"

"You mean to tell me that none of my doctors are trying to stop my cancer from spreading? And no one's trying to cure the cancer in my body?"

> **Surgery doesn't cure cancer in any way. At best, it simply removes a symptom.**

Still pacing back and forth, Dale looked at me as he spoke. "Yes, Paula, I guess I am. These may be good people, but now I realize they work in a broken system. Conventional treatments can shrink tumors, yes. They can slow down the cancer spread, yes. They can temporarily put patients into remission, yes. But conventional treatments cannot *stop* cancer from spreading. It's your immune system that destroys cancer cells—but surgery, chemo, and radiation treatments devastate your immune system."

"Dale, I feel like crying. I believe it's God's will for me to be cured, and I believe He has a plan to make that happen. But how? With all we are learning, do you think I should forget about chemotherapy or radiation? It sounds like that's what you're saying."

"Paula, we can't decide yet. We have much more to learn. But I must say we have to put the brakes on this decision until we do. If I had to choose right now based on what we've learned so far, I'd say we can't go back to conventional medicine at all. Ever. Never."

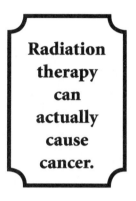

Radiation therapy can actually cause cancer.

"But my doctor said . . ." My voice trailed into silence as my thoughts took over. *Lord, my whole world is turning upside down. First the news about cancer. Then the doctors' treatment plans. And now I find out the treatments may make things worse, may even kill me. Lord, show me what to do!* I was trembling.

Dale pulled me into his arms. "Paula, I know this is a lot to take in all at once. Let's take a break."

"No. I want the truth. I *need* the truth. And I don't have time to waste. Cancer is still growing in my body. Please, go ahead. I'm ready if you're willing."

"Of course, honey. How about some good news? Did you know that thousands of people are being cured of cancer all the time—quietly, away from public view? One by one, people who commit to finding the truth and diligently search are finding ways to reverse cancer. Did you know that? I sure didn't."

"Well, that's encouraging. But why would this be one of the best kept secrets in the world? Keep talking. I'm listening."

I made myself comfortable leaning back against the bed's headboard as Dale sat down in the overstuffed chair without a pause.

"I've learned there are two camps for the treatment of

cancer: conventional medical treatment and alternative cancer treatments. Our first perception is that your doctors, and specifically your oncologist, have your interest at heart. Though they are generally wonderful people and do care about you, in reality, they don't know any way other than the conventional medical treatment. So whether it's in your best interest or not, your doctors simply aren't looking anywhere else for help.

"Paula, here's what I've come to believe. You and I personally know quite a few doctors. We also know nurses, hospital workers, and hospice care workers. Our friend Ray is a hospital administrator. And I'm certain most of these people in the medical profession sincerely want what is best for their patients. But the system is broken. It doesn't take long for man to mess up anything we get our hands on. Without God at the center, we eventually manage to make a mess of everything."

"That's right, Dale. It only makes sense that most doctors believe what they're being taught *must* be right, and what they are *not* being taught must not be very important. Don't you think? So since they're not being taught alternative cancer treatments, they must think those treatments are not important and not effective."

"Exactly. Your doctor is offering you only one path: the conventional one. Surgery, chemo, radiation. That's all they do. But many other sources claim better results from some of the alternative treatments; we've just never heard about them—until now."

"Dale, I can't believe there is so much information out there we've never heard of."

"It's shocking, isn't it? Paula, let's examine what we've learned about your options. There are conventional cancer treatments and there are alternative cancer treatments. We need to learn both sides of the issue before you make any decisions. Don't you agree?"

"Completely. It only makes sense I learn about *all* my options before deciding which way to go."

"We've talked about some of the statistics of people being cured by conventional means. We also learned the medical world calls a patient 'cured' if the cancer doesn't return within five years. But several other sources say the official numbers are skewed and in reality, only about three and a half percent are permanently cured by conventional medicine. Not only is the rate pathetically low, but it has stayed this low for over eighty years."

"Seriously? Those stats are disheartening. What do the stats for alternative medicine look like?"

"Let me get my resources on that. Hey, Paula, what do you say we go out to the porch for a change of scenery?"

"Great idea." Heading outside, I arranged two cushioned wooden chairs next to each other. The fresh air was helping me relax as I enjoyed a light breeze that wafted the scent of pine across the porch.

Soon arriving with several books and papers, Dale settled into the seat next to mine and picked up where he had left off. "Paula, an overwhelming amount of documentation reveals there are dozens of alternative treatments that *do* stop the spread of cancer—permanently. In thousands of cases, the patient has been completely cured of any signs of cancer. We're not talking remission here. We're talking cancer cure. The cancer did not return—even twenty and thirty years later. But the drug companies are not submitting these cures to the FDA. You see, natural cancer treatments don't make money for the drug companies. And successful alternative cancer treatments that *are* submitted to the FDA are labeled as 'unproven.'"

"You know, Dale, a natural cure makes sense because it's in line with God's design. I mean, since He designed our bodies to heal themselves and provided everything we would need to be healthy, where are the natural remedies? In review, a person with a healthy immune system has plenty of white blood cells that attack cancer cells and destroy them. Your research shows that it's only when the good cells can't destroy enough of the cancer cells that a person builds up a tumor. In fact, since every person gets cancer cells all the time, you have to ask yourself what causes that scale to tip out of balance?"

"That's true. It sounds funny, but I used to think cancer was a disease. Now I realize cancer isn't a disease at all! Cancer is the result of the immune system not working well enough. The real cure for cancer is found by strengthening our immune system, primarily by changing what we eat, drink, how we think, and how we live."

"Dale! Do you realize you just told me what the cure for cancer is? If I strengthen my immune system by improving what I eat, drink, how I think and live . . . it will cure me of this horrible disease. That's so logical. It's so simple. And it sounds like God."

"God knows more about cancer than the hospitals, the doctors, the chemists, and the pharmaceutical industry combined. Plus—God has integrity. He's the source of all truth. It is impossible for Him to lie. He has all the answers, and I believe He is helping us discover the truth. I don't know all I need to know about cancer yet, but we are on to something, sweetheart."

"Dale, if all this is true, then I'm going to be healed. I just know it. I'm going to be cured of cancer—permanently. And Dale, if it is true . . . if we find the answers . . . then someday . . . someday we need to write a book."

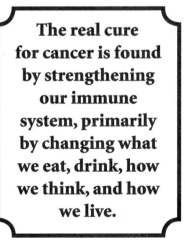

The real cure for cancer is found by strengthening our immune system, primarily by changing what we eat, drink, how we think, and how we live.

CHAPTER 11

Invisible Truth

⸻

*O*n our sixth morning in the mountains of Idyllwild, Dale and I began the day at the quaint Blue Moon Café. It had become our favorite. The food was delicious, and the atmosphere melded perfectly with the charming mountain community. The outdoor porch was dotted with a half-dozen bright blue umbrellas, offering the perfect place to enjoy the crisp mountain air. The pet-friendly environment allowed our dog, Wicket, to be leashed at our feet. My mouth watered as we placed an order for two coffees, a Denver omelet, and Dale's favorite—banana pancakes.

Relaxing moments later with our coffee, our conversation turned, as it always did, to cancer and our quest for understanding. Although most of the data we were learning was collectively unsettling, even alarming, I knew it was better to know the truth. Hiding my head in the sand because the information was hard to handle was not an option I would consider, not with cancer relentlessly spreading through my body.

Dale had previously shared with me the idea that

numerous alternative cancer treatments were available—and that thousands of patients had experienced successful results. My interest had been piqued, and I wanted to revisit the conversation. Setting my coffee down, I leaned forward.

"Dale. Why haven't we heard about these alternative methods and the successes going on all around us?"

"Well, Paula, for starters, the doctors only present the conventional treatments. There are reasons for that, some we've talked about before."

"What are some of the other reasons?"

"The best way to answer that is for me to give you a personal example because, otherwise, this could be difficult to accept."

"Okay, you've got my interest. What have we personally experienced that explains this?"

Dale turned his head away for a moment. Then, leaning forward, he raised his index finger. "Do you remember when we ran our airline pilot training business and first learned that the FAA, the NTSB, and the Airline Pilots Association are not *primarily* concerned with safety? Do you remember how hard it was to accept that truth?"

I leaned back shaking my head. "Do I? That was one of the most shocking lessons I've ever had to learn. That truth motivated us to leave the business."

"No kidding, Paula." Dale leaned back in his chair until it was balancing on the back two legs. I cringed. "We learned it firsthand—and wow, that was painful. The many forces at play are more important than passenger safety. We found that those forces have invaded labor unions, big corporations, and big government. The entire transportation industry is affected. Those forces boil down to one common denominator: money. Do you remember when we finally understood that?" Dale brought his chair back to all fours and took a long sip of coffee.

"Dale, how could I ever forget? You were a jet pilot

instructor and flight examiner for the captains on the Boeing 737. For years, we had dedicated our energies to professional training standards and aviation safety. It was devastating to learn that, when push came to shove, financial considerations trumped safety. Safety is a goal, yes, but sadly, safety is not *the* goal."

"Exactly. Paula, what I've learned about cancer has opened my eyes to the same type of perversion in the medical system. Remember John 8:32? 'And you shall know the truth, and the truth shall make you free.' Well, truth is often hard to hear, but truth *is* freeing. And regarding cancer, the truth is this: money—rather than what's best for the patient—rules. And that's the truth."

"I suppose that shouldn't surprise me." I leaned forward. "But what makes you so sure of it?"

"Well, I've learned there's an unholy alliance between the pharmaceutical industry and the FDA. The FDA constantly approves drugs—not necessarily because they're helpful to the patient but because they bring in money and profits to the huge pharmaceutical industry. True, some of the drugs *extend* the life of cancer patients—but none of them cure cancer." Dale leaned forward and gently grabbed my arm. "Paula, as I've told you, I'm learning that cancer *is* curable, even reversible."

"But, Dale, are you sure? If there's a cure, why wouldn't the medical system be jumping all over it?"

Dale squeezed my wrist tighter and lowered his voice to a whisper. "The medical industry doesn't *want* to cure cancer. The industry would lose too much money, too many jobs, and too much power."

"I don't think I want to believe that, Dale."

"I know, sweetheart. Neither do I." Dale released my wrist. "But, Paula, it's true. I read an article by a medical doctor who claimed the American Medical Association is nothing more than a giant labor union and has never approved a procedure that can stop the spread of cancer. Even some orthodox cancer treatments have been shut down by the authorities—usually the AMA, the FDA, or the FTC—because they were far too effective in curing people of the disease. Can you believe that?"

I didn't think I could feel any lower. But I was wrong.

For a moment, Dale lowered his head. "The reality, Paula, is that extending the life of people with cancer makes more money than curing them." He leaned back in his chair. "Think about it. Doesn't the Bible say that the love of money is the root of all evil?"

"But, Dale, how can patients be allowed to die because of greed? That would be murder." Dale slowly nodded and sipped his coffee. I wanted to jump up in frustration and anger. It was almost too much to contemplate . . . and yet it rang true. Deep down, I knew it made sense. It was consistent with what I knew about big business, about how the world often worked. I hated to think about the negative side of things, but my life was on the line. I couldn't afford to be naive.

The food arrived and we ate, mostly in silence. The good mood of the morning and the quaint atmosphere of the Blue Moon Café had been lost in the face of what Dale was telling me about the medical industry. Even the food now seemed tasteless.

Leaving some bills on the table to cover the check, Dale asked, "Paula, do you think you could take a short walk?"

"Yes, I need to, Dale. I'm so stressed, but I'm not sure how far I'll be able to go. My side is really hurting." Leaving the café, we gingerly trekked about a hundred yards. By then, the pain was too much. I leaned on Dale's arm and we circled back to the car, Wicket in tow. I couldn't tell if the short walk actually relieved my stress or caused more. But during that time, I made a solemn and silent proclamation: *I will not come off this mountain without finding my way of escape! I will not!*

Back at the cabin, we gathered several books we had been

studying and carried them outdoors to the front porch to continue our discussion. With the fresh air, nature's view, a glass of iced tea, and my newfound resolve, I began to feel better.

Dale jumped right in. "Paula, do you realize over many decades there have been multiple opportunities to cure cancer, but the cure has been held back every time? Why? Because of money. Profits. It is far more profitable to *slow* the spread of cancer than to stop it.

"You see, if they find the cure for cancer, our medical system would lose literally billions of dollars every year. Hundreds of thousands of jobs would disappear—not just in the medical field but in all cancer related fields. But if they can keep cancer as a chronic disease, it provides a long-term profit machine. The truth can be heartbreaking, can't it?"

"Dale, this is completely gut-wrenching. But you know, as hard as this is to believe, the more I think about it, the more believable it becomes—especially after personally experiencing something so similar in the aviation industry."

"Paula, your indignation is well-founded. If you put the American Cancer Society, the National Cancer Institute, and the American Medical Association together, they provide a fertile environment of control. They are literally one of the largest moneymaking organizations in the world. And money means power. These three powerhouses of the medical industry are controlling what treatments are offered within the medical system. Cancer has become big business."

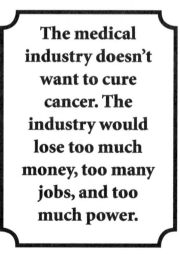

The medical industry doesn't want to cure cancer. The industry would lose too much money, too many jobs, and too much power.

Dale stood and leaned against the wooden railing. Facing me and trying not to sound too upset he continued, "I've been doing research on the big pharmaceutical companies too. They regularly develop new and different prescription drugs for all kinds of diseases. But better for whom? Hardly ever better for the patient. Like in all business, the main goal is to increase profits. It doesn't matter that many of these drugs are toxic and even deadly. It's about the bottom line—protect shareholder profits!

"And then we see these drugs advertised on television and radio and in medical journals—and in magazines and promotional literature. I've learned that in many cases, there's little scientific evidence that these drugs are actually beneficial. The public is conditioned to believe *new and better* drugs are the answer to our medical problems, but that is seldom the case. In fact, because the test groups are so limited, we wait to discover the results of these new drugs—like guinea pigs in a giant lab."

"Dale, I'm shocked to hear how broken our medical system really is."

"I know, Paula. These pharmaceutical corporations wield powerful influence in ways I had never imagined." Dale picked up a book and opened it to a paper-clipped page. "In this book, *Dissent in Medicine: Nine Doctors Speak Out,* Dr. Alan Levin describes how the drug companies entertain physicians with elaborate dinners and parties. And how they fund the building of hospitals, medical schools, and research facilities. Most shockingly, discussing the effectiveness—or ineffectiveness— of chemotherapy, Dr. Levin says, 'Most physicians agree that chemotherapy is largely ineffective for the majority of cancers. Despite this fact, honest physicians are coerced into using these treatment modalities by special interest groups who have a vested interest in the profits of the drug industry.'[21] Paula, isn't this staggering, that a doctor would make these public indictments against the drug companies?

"Now listen to this." Dale thumbed through his stack of

notes and print-offs. "Author Mike Adams, a well-respected health and nutrition guru, wrote, 'It is not an exaggeration to call this a medical holocaust. These drug companies seem determined to dose the entire population with as many simultaneous prescriptions as possible, as long as it generates profits for their shareholders. Business ethics are nowhere to be found in the pharmaceutical industry these days: it's all about money, profits, power and control.'"[22]

Pulling a prescription bottle from my purse, I stared at it in disdain, then shoved it back into my purse.

Dale continued, "Here's something else Mike Adams wrote: 'Doctors who prescribed the drug company's products and avoided competing drugs were paid "consulting fees" of tens of thousands of dollars' and 'Doctors were paid even more money to conduct fraudulent clinical trials.'[23] Isn't that unbelievable, Paula?"

"Dale, this is scary stuff. It's difficult to accept, but I believe it."

"There's more; listen to this." Dale shuffled through his papers until he found the one he wanted. "In July 2004, Dr. Marcia Angell, physician, as well as former editor-in-chief of the *New England Journal of Medicine* for over twenty years, wrote an article called 'The Truth About the Drug Companies.' She said this about the pharmaceutical industry: 'Now, primarily a marketing machine to sell drugs of dubious benefit, this industry uses its wealth and power to co-opt every institution that might stand in its way, including the United States Congress, the FDA, academic medical centers, and the medical profession itself.' She went on to say that unfortunately there are no checks and balances on this industry or its quest for profits. One of the most shocking facts in 2002 was that the combined profits of the new drug companies in the Fortune 500 (almost thirty-six billion) were more than the profits for all the other 490 businesses put together (less than thirty-four billion).[24]

"Then there is Webster Kehr, Chairman of the Independent Cancer Research Foundation, Inc. He describes the approach of the pharmaceutical industry: 'Find a natural substance that cures something, bury this fact, then fabricate, synthesize, and mutate the key natural substance, then patent the mutation, and make huge profits.' Paula, I'm beginning to understand that because the pharmaceutical companies can't patent or profit from natural remedies, they change what they can into a man-made synthetic form in order to sell it."[25]

"That's a complete perversion of God's design for natural healing."

"That's exactly what it is. But listen, Paula, I have some good news too. Let me share some statistics I learned about alternative treatments. They're pretty exciting."

"Oh, Dale, yes. Please. I could use some good news."

> **Pursuing the right alternative approach first provides the best opportunity for the patient to experience a reversal of cancer and ultimately a permanent cure.**

"The stats I'm going to be talking about are the kind that people stick their names to and stake their careers on."

"Great. I love it. Tell me more."

"Okay, here goes. According to several studies, a true cancer cure of at least ninety percent *can* be accomplished *if* the cancer patient does several things. They must turn to the right alternative treatment first, not last. It's important to avoid orthodox or conventional treatments and, instead, use one of the many successful alternative methods and follow it diligently. They must do their homework and make the necessary changes in what they eat, what they drink, how they think, and how they live. Pursuing the right alternative approach *first* provides the best opportunity for the patient to experience a reversal of cancer and ultimately a permanent cure. Ninety percent, Paula. That's certainly different from the average of the three percent who use conventional medicine to survive to the magic five-year mark!"

"You're right; those are really encouraging studies and much better statistics."

"But listen to this. Ninety-five percent of cancer patients who use some form of alternative cancer treatment have *already* had conventional treatments. That's almost everyone. Many of them had everything orthodox medicine could offer and were sent home to die. This means the alternative medicine was chosen as a last resort when they were already in dire critical condition and medical science had given up on them."

"And did alternative methods work for any of those who had already done conventional treatments?"

"Absolutely, yes. I've learned that it's critical to *start* with an alternative treatment instead of end with one. Unfortunately, there are only a small handful of alternative treatments strong enough to help after chemo and radiation have done their damage. Still, amazingly, fifty percent of those who were sent home to die after conventional medicine failed them found a cure for their cancer by turning to an effective alternative treatment. Fifty percent!"

"That's fantastic! So how many different kinds of alternative cancer treatments are there?"

"There are hundreds, Paula. And we're going to learn all about the most successful ones. I think we're going to find something that will be right for you, crystal clear, and one-hundred percent successful."

"This is getting exciting."

"It really is. God is showing us truth, and the truth is going to make us free—make you cancer free, Paula. I believe that with all my heart."

My eyes teared up. "Dale, we're learning so much more than I even knew existed. The mysteries of cancer are beginning to fade. To be uncovering such huge truths in just a few days of research is mind-boggling. God is helping us find what we need."

Smiling, Dale lifted his glass. In a pitiful Humphrey Bogart delivery, he murmured, "Here's looking at you, kid."

I grinned. My stomach filled with butterflies.

Hope was taking root.

CHAPTER 12

Hiding in Plain Sight

*D*ale and I remained on the porch, sipping iced teas and quietly sifting through our treasure trove of data. The silence was occasionally interrupted by exclamations of discovery. With each new find, the cancer puzzle was forming a clearer picture. A picture that looked nothing at all like what we had expected when our journey began.

It was only a matter of time before Dale threw out another bomb. "Paula, listen to this. This is another quote from *World Without Cancer: The Story of Vitamin B-17* by G. Edward Griffin: 'With billions of dollars spent each year in research, with additional billions taken in from the cancer related sale of drugs, and with the vote-hungry politicians promising ever-increasing government programs, today, there are more people making a living from cancer than dying from it.'[26]

"This guy talks about the *politics* of cancer being way more complex than the science of cancer. He attributes this to the fact that if there were a cure to this horrid disease, the entire commercial and political industry of cancer would be erased overnight. And that isn't going to happen."

"Oh my gosh, Dale. It feels like a lost cause. Even the well-meaning people who donate toward the cure through fundraising races and events are just feeding the monster more of what it's after . . . money and power."

> "The cancer industry survives and thrives by perpetually searching for the cure but never finding it."
>
> — Ty Bollinger

"I'm sure you're right, Paula. Every dollar that comes in only feeds an insatiable appetite for more. Here's a book called *Cancer: Step Outside the Box.* It was written by a bestselling author and a cancer cure advocate." Dale opened the book to a paper-clipped page. "Ty Bollinger writes, 'The cancer industry survives and thrives by perpetually searching for the cure but never finding it. . . . The cancer industry is perpetuating lies and fraud. This fraud is of unspeakable magnitude.'"[27]

*So many lives lost . . ."*Wow, that's a strong statement, Dale. I'm not completely sold yet, but there's so much evidence when you start looking. And after hearing what you said about the pharmaceutical industry, I did my own research and found some other stats and information. Want to hear what I found?"

"Absolutely. Go ahead, Paula, tell me."

"The pharmaceutical companies now spend eighteen and a half billion dollars every year promoting their drugs just to physicians. Did you hear that? Gosh, that amounts to about thirty-thousand dollars per year per physician in just the United States alone. That is unconscionable.

"Now I think we're getting a better picture of what's going on. No wonder the truth is being suppressed. Apparently, it *is* about the money. The conventional treatments are being pushed on the public and the natural remedies, the ones that actually *stop* cancer, are relegated to the background—even hidden from the people who need them."

Dale and I sat for a while, listening to the wind through the pines, contemplating the magnitude of what we were uncovering.

At last, shaking his head, Dale broke the silence. "Paula, the doctors, the oncologists—none of them are administering anything that cures cancer. Their synthetic drugs and medical procedures do nothing to keep cancer from spreading. No one in conventional medicine is dealing with the root cause of the disease—they're only dealing with symptoms. I believe many doctors want to cure their patients, but there's an abundance of evidence that the industry doesn't share that goal."

"Considering what we're learning, I have to agree with you, Dale. The medical industry as a whole doesn't seem to *want* a cure for cancer."

"Even the doctors are kept in the dark. I think if you gave most doctors who are treating cancer patients all these statistics, they'd have trouble believing them. They simply aren't taught about alternative treatments or their successes. Doctors believe that if alternative methods worked, they'd have learned about them in medical school or read about them in the medical journals. But since medical schools are almost entirely funded by large pharmaceutical companies, and other organizations with a vested interest in conventional cancer treatments, the doctors aren't getting any competing information."

Dale, rigid with frustration, blurted out, "And why would any doctors do their own independent research? Why would doctors want to learn what we're learning? It would go cross-grain with everything the industry believes and practices. Burying their head, taking the money and lavish perks, having favor with peers—all these benefits far outweigh the alternative of knowing the truth . . . and becoming an outcast in their profession."

"I know, Dale. The more people who have cancer, the more money goes into the medical system. A lot of livelihoods and careers depend on the continuation of cancer treatment. It's becoming clear that money instead of morals is the guiding light for the cancer industry."

"If the doctors treat the symptoms but never address the root cause, the medical machinery keeps spinning. Listen to this, Paula." Riffling through his notes, Dale found the desired page and read aloud, "The war on cancer was declared officially in 1971 by the federal government of the United States when President Richard Nixon signed Senate Bill 1828, called the National Cancer Act of 1971.[28] Since then more than two trillion dollars have been spent on cancer research and conventional cancer treatments. But is the cancer treatment getting better results? No. According to the statistics, it's getting worse."

"Dale, how can curing cancer cost more and take more time than going to the moon?"

"I know the answer to that one, Paula. It can't. It cost between twenty to twenty-five billion dollars for all the Apollo missions, before and including the moon mission in 1969."

"That's what I'm talking about, Dale. I'm having trouble believing it's more difficult for the cancer industry to find a cure for cancer than it was for science to find a way to go to the moon. But why would the industry want to find a cure when it's so lucrative not to?"

Dale's shoulders slumped. "Of course, you're right. And listen to this. Dr. John Bailar, who was an editor of the *Journal of the National Cancer Institute* and worked for the cancer institute for twenty-five years, spoke at the American Association for the Advancement of Science. Do you know what he said? 'My overall assessment is that the national cancer program must be judged a qualified failure.'[29]

"I've said it before, but let me say it again. Paula, when it comes to treating chronic disease, keep me out of the hospital. Sure, we need hospitals for broken bones, accidents, things like that. But for treating disease or chronic illness—hospitals are a death trap."

My head was spinning. It seemed we had opened Pandora's Box. We were discovering hidden evils that had always been right under our noses.

"There's a pattern I'm seeing, Dale. In the medical system, at least here in the U.S., if something is found that works naturally—something that cannot be patented—it is removed from public view as quickly as possible and discredited as ineffective. At the same time, incredibly dangerous and ineffective synthetic drugs are routinely approved by the FDA and prescribed for the public. The general population naively trusts its doctors, the FDA, and the medical system. The public is kept at arm's length from the facts and remains largely ignorant of the truth."

"Paula, I think we're looking at one of the largest deceptions in U.S. history. This just sickens me. I've never seen a bigger fraud in my life. It's almost impossible to believe, but truth often is." Dale flipped open another book. "Listen to this from Dr. Linus Pauling—this guy was a two-time Nobel prizewinner and is regarded as one of the most important scientists of the twentieth century. He said, 'Most cancer research is largely a fraud, and the major cancer research organizations are derelict in their duties to the people who

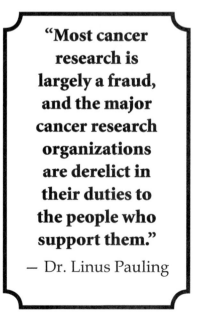

"Most cancer research is largely a fraud, and the major cancer research organizations are derelict in their duties to the people who support them."

— Dr. Linus Pauling

support them.'[30] Paula, this is coming from a *two-time Nobel prizewinner*."

"That's despicable, Dale. The faces of all the people we've known who have died of cancer keep scrolling through my mind. What a tragic waste of human life. Although I'm gaining hope in what we're discovering, it's making me sick to my stomach at the same time."

Inspired by the moment, Dale leaned forward and took my hands. "Paula, let me suggest we do something right now that we've never done before. Let's take fifteen minutes, no more and no less, and write down the names of those we have known closely who died of cancer. You know, friends and family—not just acquaintances. Let's reflect on how this cancer fraud has affected our lives and how many loved ones we've lost because of this maddening pack of lies."

"Dale, that's a good idea. I want to know how big this tragedy is and how dramatically it has impacted us personally."

For precisely fifteen minutes, Dale and I sat in silence, writing down names of those we'd lost to cancer. The lists kept growing. We thought back through the years, recalling cherished loved ones who were no longer a part of our lives. With each departure, we had lost a piece of our hearts. I began feeling the loss of these precious loved ones all over again. Seeing Dale slowly shaking his drooped head, I could tell he felt the same.

At the end of fifteen minutes, we compared our lists and tallied up the numbers: eleven family members had succumbed to cancer—from grandparents to aunts and uncles and cousins. We also remembered twenty-eight close friends, roommates, college friends, people we had vacationed with, close friends from church, missionaries and pastors we'd worked with side by side, and airline pilots Dale had flown with. The total number was stunning: thirty-nine. Thirty-nine precious family and friends whose lives had been cut short by cancer. And if we included our acquaintances who had died from this dreadful disease, that number almost tripled. I could barely breathe. Dale and I needed a break. The gut-wrenching exercise had rekindled my grief and anguish. Further fueled by the lies we were uncovering, my emotions quickly ignited into anger.

"Would you like to take a walk up the street and back?" Dale asked.

"I don't think so. My abdomen is hurting too much right now . . . I wouldn't get very far. Why don't you go on without me?" Fear had been progressively tightening my chest. I welcomed a few minutes to myself to wrestle with the single thought that dominated my mind: *My name cannot be added to the list. Please, God, spare me that fate.*

Leaving to work off his stress alone, Dale headed down the porch steps growling, "I'll be back."

Twenty minutes later, Dale returned and slumped down in a chair. I could see he was visibly shaken. After giving him a couple of moments to gain his composure, I asked, "Are you going to be alright, honey? What happened?"

He exhaled and dropped his head, releasing some internal tension. "While I was taking my walk, I remembered several more people who died of cancer who we forgot to put on our list."

"What?" *How could there be more?* "Like who?"

For a few moments I listened to Dale recite more names, and with each name, a face and personal history flashed across my mind. *How could we have forgotten them?* Each represented extended family or a friend neither of us had recalled during our allotted fifteen-minute exercise, yet these were people we loved and shared our lives with. How could we have forgotten them? I felt ashamed—guilty.

Even before I was diagnosed, cancer had *already* devastated our lives. And not only ours, but the family members of each person whose life had been snuffed out prematurely. Dale and I reeled. *How many more would we remember in the days ahead?* It was all too much. I needed hope—and I needed more answers. Now. "Dale, tell me about the alternative treatments. Are they working? And if they are, why aren't more people using them?"

"Well, Paula, I've only recently begun researching the alternative treatments. But already one of the lies I've been finding in the medical literature is that there is no good evidence that any alternative treatment can prevent cancer. Think about that. That is exactly what the people we know seem to believe. That's even what *we* thought until this week. Countless good people believe that alternative treatment is unproven and therefore is most likely a scam. They believe that if the doctors don't tell you about it, it can't be valid. No doubt, most doctors are unaware of the research that's been going on for an entire century and shows tremendous help for curing cancer—and many other diseases for that matter."

"I don't think most doctors know about other options, Dale. I found statistics from a study carried out by the Institute for Evidence-Based Medicine in Germany. They found that ninety-four percent of the information contained in promotional literature sent to doctors has no scientific basis whatsoever. None. Now that's shocking. But if the doctors believe the medical literature, then it's really not that surprising that they aren't open to other choices."

"That's so true, Paula. What do you say we take a break and head inside for some sandwiches and more iced tea? I'm ready for something to eat. And my brain could use the recess."

Lunch was a much needed diversion from our heavy conversation on the porch. But true to form, as soon as we finished our meal, we picked up our conversation right where we had left off.

"Paula, not only does the medical establishment suppress

information about alternative cancer treatments—I've also learned about people being persecuted for promoting alternative treatments. There are even documented cases of murder."

"Are you kidding? That sounds pretty extreme. Dale, you aren't one to believe wild accusations."

"I know . . . you're right. But I've uncovered a lot of credible documentation about these cases. I've been reading example after example where a person's character is attacked and their reputation ruined. Paula, doctors and scientists who are learning the truth about cancer and other chronic diseases and treating these diseases with natural remedies are being persecuted and suppressed even in our own country. They are being completely discredited. For years, hundreds of very concerned and conscientious health providers and herbalists who have been using alternative methods have been treated like criminals."

"Like who? Can you give me any examples?"

For the next two hours, Dale sat across the kitchen table and read statistics and facts documenting how eleven major doctors were persecuted and how their healing information was suppressed. "The most notable one to me was Dr. Max Gerson, a German Jewish medical doctor who came to the United States just before World War II. He documented evidence of curing multiple terminal cancer patients as well as patients with tuberculosis and other diseases. He wrote a book describing fifty cancer patients and their cures. But Gerson was literally poisoned to death—murdered because his treatments were outside the establishment's accepted protocol. Dr. Gerson's treatments were all natural and highly successful."

As Dale shared these cases and I saw the documentation with my own eyes, he convinced me that the most effective alternative cancer treatments over the past century have been lost or suppressed. Records were destroyed, offices ransacked, and people were persecuted and silenced.

"Paula, Satan is behind all of this—that's clear. When people quit thinking for themselves and don't challenge what they're being told, they become easy prey for the enemy. What does the Bible say Satan has come to do?"

"Steal, kill, and destroy. Dale, we can sure see him at work in the cancer industry."

"Exactly. And remember this scripture? 'Your adversary the devil walks about like a roaring lion, seeking whom he may devour.'[31] Well, that's the medical system, including pharmaceutical companies that do major marketing for their conventional treatments. At the same time, they tell people the alternative approach is not effective at best, or is fraud at worst."

"Dale, I think we're conditioned to believe almost anything as long as we trust the source. Unfortunately, conventional medical treatments have been legitimized by their massive use. It's amazing to learn that the real cause of cancer is already known. I read a scientific explanation of what cancer *really* is—and

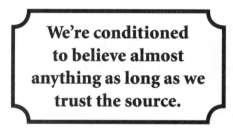

We're conditioned to believe almost anything as long as we trust the source.

knowing what it is allows it to be reversed. And because they can't cure it with surgery, chemo, and radiation, they keep the truth clouded in a sea of mystery."

"Paula, the reality is, if you're not a drug company and not FDA approved—another hornet's nest—you can't make health claims about your product in the United States. It doesn't matter if your claims are documented and supported by studies. But if you are a drug company, you can buy your researchers and pay for fabricated data. In my opinion, the FDA is not primarily concerned with truth—or health. The FDA seems to be protecting the profits of the drug companies. I know that's hard to believe, but when you look at the facts, it becomes clear. The public has a misguided and false sense of security. There is a grand deception going on, and it's about hiding the cure for cancer."

Dale picked up another book and thumbed to a specific page. "Paula, this one is earth-shattering to me. Here's an article about the hypocrisy of the FDA. We think they're here to protect us, but that no longer seems to be the case. According to Congresswoman Louise Slaughter, 'It's shameful that the FDA has abandoned its responsibility to protect the health and safety of Americans in favor of protecting an industry it is supposed to be regulating.' She goes on to state that 'if the FDA would put as much effort into fulfilling their mandate to protect the public's health as they do into their pro-industry media campaign, we might start to make some headway.'[32] And, Paula, it's apparently been like this for years.

"Way back in 1970, former FDA Commissioner Dr. Herbert Ley said, 'People think the FDA is protecting them. It is not. What the FDA is doing and what the public thinks it's doing are as different as night and day.'"[33]

Dale continued, "In his book *FDA, You Were Wrong!* Dr. Robert W. Christensen disclosed the following about his dealings with the FDA. He said there are '. . . conflicts of interest, lying, cover-up and other possibly criminal behavior of persons within the Food and Drug Administration.'[34] He goes on to state that 'unfair, destructive

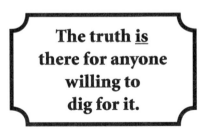

The truth <u>is</u> there for anyone willing to dig for it.

practices and overregulation have stopped innovation, thus stopping America.' These are credible people who recognize the hypocritical deficiency of the FDA.

"Paula, this entire deception is rooted in what I call

'marketing mania.' People stop thinking for themselves and believe whatever they are told or whatever they read—as long as it's from the established system. The medical industry can't afford to let the truth out. But the truth *is* there for anyone willing to dig for it."

I stood and placed my hand on Dale's shoulder. "Thanks for all your help, honey. In learning about cancer, we've come a long way. One thing has become abundantly clear throughout this process: There *is* truth to be found. And in this journey, step by step, my hope is growing. Still, we need to keep digging because, Dale . . . I'm running out of time."

CHAPTER 13

I Found It!

⌒

Morning dawned bright and clear, the sunlight wrestling around the trees to make its way through the large windows. My feelings of hope from the night before had grown even stronger, and I was more determined than ever to stay the course . . . to keep digging until I found my way of escape.

Laden with sweet rolls, fresh orange juice, and hot coffee, Dale and I trekked to the cabin's sunny front porch with Wicket trailing at our heels. Our seventh day got underway with a delightful breakfast and a serenade of clamorous mountain blue jays. Once the pot of coffee ran dry, we headed back inside and readied ourselves to dive back into the sea of information.

Gathering the books we had yet to read and spreading them out on the king-sized bed, I scanned and reviewed each one for the next couple of hours, evaluating their content. Several told the stories of people who shared their journey, only to die in the end. Others, written by a spouse or family member, wrote about acts of courage and inspiration of a loved one who ultimately succumbed to the disease. I was left with a sinking, sickening feeling in my stomach. The hope that had been growing in recent days began to wilt, threatening to disappear completely. *Will I find my answer in one of these remaining books? Or will I learn all this information and work enormously hard, only to die like the people I've read about?*

It was time for a change. I needed to talk.

Dale was bent over the coffee table writing notes from an open paperback. Checking his watch as he raised his head, he asked, "What's up? Are you ready for a break?"

"No, it's not that, Dale. I'm finding two very different types of books. Many of them are about people who died from cancer—I don't want to read those. I want to live, Dale." I tried not to sound desperate. "I need to read about successes, not failures. Some of the books are about people who got well— those are the ones I need. I want to know *how* they got well. Then there are the ones with statistics, facts, and information. How can we narrow down the number of books we're dealing with? There are just too many and not enough time!"

"Okay, sweetheart, I can see your problem. That's a valid issue," Dale concurred, setting down his pen and pushing aside his notes. "Why don't we take a break on the back porch?"

I poured us each a fresh glass of iced tea, which we carried outside. Standing against the redwood railing and breathing the crisp clean air helped clear my emotions and buoyed my spirit. We were both silent for a few moments. I smiled at two squirrels quarreling in an adjacent pine. *This break was a good idea.*

Sipping on his tea, Dale turned. "Paula, why don't we sort all the books into three categories? The first group will be books about people who got well and lived. The second pile can be about people who died. You're right—we need to stay away from those. And the third pile can be neutral . . . you know, facts and information and stuff like that. Tell me about the package you got from your mom. What's in that?"

"Two video tapes and a workbook. But there's no VCR player in the cabin. I guess I'll have to wait until we get home to see them."

"Well, Paula, there's a good chance we could rent a player here in Idyllwild. Would you like me to try?"

"Sure, that would be great. I'm really anxious to see why Mom was so inspired to send them to me."

"Okay. I'll see if I can pick one up next time we're in town."

We headed back inside and proceeded to divide the books, categorizing them into stacks. We labeled the first group "Life," the next pile, "Death." Last, we grouped the books on "Data" and "How-Tos," which we integrated with the "Life" pile. Once we had finished the process, Dale scooped up the "Death" books, walked them outside, and swiftly dumped them into the trunk of the car. I'd never see them again.

Dale strode back into the cabin, closing the front door. Ever the encourager, he smiled, "Don't forget, Paula, you're going to get well. God's will is that you are healed. The entire family is praying that way. You *will* get well, honey. Your healing *is* God's will, you know."

"I know it is, Dale, but so many things that are God's will don't turn out the way He wants them to. I see good people die all the time from sickness and accidents. According to the Bible, that is not God's will—yet it happens anyway."

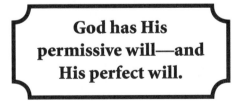

God has His permissive will—and His perfect will.

"That's true. But let's not forget that God has His *permissive* will—and His *perfect* will. We've both learned there's more to it than just *knowing* God's will. You can *know* the speed limit, yet choose to violate it—and suffer the consequences. Speaking as a pilot, I can know about gravity, ignore that law, and suffer dire repercussions. Or you can have something happen to you that you didn't choose or even know about, but it still happened and you have to deal with the results.

"Paula, cancer has invaded your body. We don't yet know why or how we're going to combat this, but we *will* find out. There are laws of cause and effect. And let me tell you—no, let me promise you—if there *is* a cause of cancer, we're going to discover that cause. Then we'll figure out how to reverse it. As you know, finding the cause of a problem is usually half the battle. God promised you a way of escape—and that agrees with His will for you to get well. So now it's up to us to seek the method and develop our faith for a successful outcome. It is *not* His *perfect* will for anyone to die of sickness, yet many do within His *permissive* will. He promised you a way of escape— now we're going to do our part. We'll move heaven and earth if we have to until we find it."

Dale's optimism was rubbing off. "Thank you for that, Dale. It really helps."

Suddenly a Bible parable came to mind. "You know, Dale, it makes me think about the parable Jesus taught about the one lost sheep. The shepherd left the ninety-nine sheep to search for the one that was lost. And he searched *until* he found it.[35] The shepherd didn't just stay with the flock and pray. He didn't look a little while and give up. He searched as long as it took. He *did* something. He took action and kept at it until he found what he was looking for. That's what I'm going to do—search until I find my answer . . . God's way of escape for me."

"Awesome, Paula." Dale wiped a tear and smiled. "Then back to work. We still have a lot of data to wade through. And we need to spend as much time in prayer as we do in research—agreed?"

"Absolutely," I called back, surprised at the enthusiasm in my own voice. "I'll see you again in a couple of hours."

Statistics, recommended treatments, types of cancer, side effects, and survival rates. The subjects were endless. My head was swimming. *How can the medical profession know so much about cancer and everything that goes with it, yet know so little about why people get cancer and how to get rid of it?*

Looking deeper, I became distraught when I learned how many people survived for several years only to end up with cancer again—the disease often fatal the second time. The survival statistics were disheartening. *Lord, I feel like a yo-yo. My hope starts building—and then it drains away as I read all this discouraging information.*

Dr. Anderson's words still rang in my ears. "If you do nothing more, you'll not be alive in three to six months." The afternoon was over in a flash and my mind was spent. *Just how much information can one person cram into her brain in one day?* It was time for a recess.

Dale and I drove down the winding road toward town for dinner. It was relaxing to breathe the fresh air and let my mind wander for a while. Several squirrels raced across the road like miniature daredevils, barely missing our car. We stopped at a roadside hamburger joint that boasted the best burgers on the hill. Dale found seats outside while I went back to the car to retrieve a sweater. The evening breeze had kicked in and the temperatures were cooling quickly.

When I arrived at the table, Dale looked up and mumbled in a pitiful Humphrey Bogart voice, "Of all the hamburger joints in all the towns in all the world, you had to walk into mine."

I sat down with a smile, shaking my head. Ignoring his woeful attempt to lighten the mood, I asked, "Dale, can we try to get a little more done this evening after dinner? We have only a few days before we head home and I still haven't found my answer." I pushed down the panicky feelings. "Gosh, I'm being worn out

LIFE, CANCER AND GOD

by this up and down emotional roller coaster. One moment I'm up, feeling full of faith, and the next I'm sinking into despair. Hope goes out the window when I read about those who have died or think about all the people I knew who died of cancer. Not only that, but my physical symptoms are getting worse. Every time I feel pain in my abdomen or notice the lump on my arm, panic sets in. I need to find my answer soon."

"Believe it or not sweetheart, I completely understand. I went through a similar roller coaster in the aftermath of the airplane crash. You're in the middle of a large storm, more like a hurricane."

"I know you're right. But I've never been diagnosed with cancer before. Never looked so closely into death's eye. Never had a doctor tell me I could be dead in a few months—and that was over a month ago. Is there anything you can say that might help? I can't seem to stabilize my faith."

"I think what you're going through has to do with the difference between hope and faith. You've diligently studied God's Word all of your adult life . . . so let's review what we know. Remember, Paula, hope and faith are like twins but they're not the same. Hope is the blueprint of faith. And faith is the evidence of things you believe in—but are not yet seen.

> **Hope and faith are like twins, but they're not the same. Hope is the blueprint of faith. Faith is the evidence of things you believe in but don't see.**

"When a builder constructs a building, he references the blueprints before and during the building process. Hope is that blueprint. It is believing in something that is still 'out there.' You don't *have* it yet, but you *hope* for it. You want it and believe it will be yours someday . . . but it's still out there in the future.

146

"Then there's faith. The Bible says that faith is the substance of things hoped for, the evidence of things not seen.[36] Faith is when you take hold of something you hope for. You *grab* it and pull it into the *here and now.* It has not manifested—is not visible yet. But faith seizes what you hope for and brings it into the present. First, you hope for it. But with faith in your heart, it feels and appears as if it has already arrived in the here and now. When you have real faith, then as far as you're concerned, what you were hoping for has already happened."

> As God's Word goes deep into your heart and you believe it, speak it, act on it, and live as if it's true—that's when it becomes faith.

"Dale, I understand that I'm hoping God will heal me or show me how to get well. I'm trusting in the promise He gave me, that He will provide a way of escape from this horrible disease . . . and from death. But I can't seem to hold onto faith."

"Paula, you've found hope in God's Word that He wants you well. And there's no place you can ever establish faith other than God's Word. The Bible scripture always has to be the starting line. But you have to keep going—praying, searching, and striving for God's will to be accomplished. As you get God's Word deep into your heart and believe it, speak it, act on it, and live as if it's true—that's when it becomes faith. And that faith is what opens the door to receiving what you are believing for."

After dinner we headed over to the video store, where Dale was able to rent a VCR player. Arriving back at the cabin just as the sun dipped behind the top of the mountains, we prepared to tackle our project once more. I was eager to check out the videos Mom sent. Dale hooked up the VCR to the TV in the master bedroom, and I popped in the tape as he headed back to the living room to continue his research.

An attractive woman appeared on the screen. She was a medical doctor who had been diagnosed with advanced, stage IV breast cancer. As a doctor, she had access to the best medical help money could buy. Yet, she chose *not* to use the medical system to treat her cancer. *Fascinating!*

Dr. Kay Cohen more than understood the protocol for cancer treatment but chose to reject surgery, chemo, and radiation. In her desperation, she turned to God for the first time in her life and became a new Christian. Then she began searching for a natural cure—ultimately finding a way to completely reverse her cancer. Although she used different words, I knew immediately that she had used the body, soul, and spirit approach that Dale and I had been discovering for several weeks.

My eyes were riveted to the screen. Dr. Cohen's every word burned into my heart. The truths she was sharing were confirming many of the things I had been recently learning. God was using this woman—a medical doctor—to pull it all together in a concise and usable way. Excitement welled in me until I could hardly contain it. Dots connected and critical pieces of the cancer puzzle fell into place at lightning speed.

Dr. Cohen's alternative treatment plan eventually worked, and she became cancer free. Her tumor had been huge, yet gradually disappeared while following her newly discovered alternative path.

By the time the tape ended, I could barely breathe. For a while, I just sat and stared at the blank screen, my heart doing summersaults. I sensed the same electrifying feeling I had when God first promised me a way of escape. *This was it!*

I jumped up, grabbed the tape from the machine, and ran into the living room waving it above my head. "I found it! Dale, I found it!"

"What? What's wrong, Paula?" Dale looked up, startled.

"Nothing's wrong. Everything is right." My heart pounded in my chest. Still waving the tape I hollered, "I found it, Dale . . . I found my way of escape!"

CHAPTER 14

Mountain Chaos

Our respite in the mountains was quickly coming to a close—we would be leaving early the next morning. I had spent the previous three days devouring all of Dr. Cohen's materials in preparation for implementing a natural alternative plan for reversing the cancer spreading in my body.

My mind, already gorged with much heart-stirring information, was striving to absorb even more. But soon I would need to do more than learn—I would need to take action. Time was running out, and it was critical that I start implementing radical changes. The spiritual insights and truths Dale and I had tried and tested throughout the years provided a solid foundation. Now, adding the natural healing principles Dr. Cohen was sharing about the body would dramatically enhance my arsenal for waging war against cancer. My Body-Soul-Spirit approach was rapidly taking shape.

We had spent much of the morning cleaning the cabin in preparation for the next day's departure. Dale had made a final run into town to return the video player, call home for phone messages, and pick up fresh carrot juice. I reclined on the shady front porch with Wicket at my feet, reviewing my list of to-dos. The intense requirements of my new lifestyle, including juicing ten times daily, would be all consuming once I returned home. My life was about to change again—dramatically.

My thoughts drifted to what I'd been learning. Though Dale supported my commitment to this new alternative anti-cancer regimen, he felt it would be best not to put all our eggs in one basket. He would continue to research other successful alternatives. By studying the Gerson Therapy, Dr. Lorraine Day's Natural Health Plan, and about a dozen other approaches, we both felt we wouldn't be leaving any stone unturned.

Enjoying a few moments of peaceful solitude, I leaned my head back and relaxed. The mountain chatter of squirrels and blue jays filled the air. But then suddenly, the screaming engine of a car intruded. I could hear it long before it came into view. It was our car, and it was racing up the hill toward the cabin at breakneck speed. *Something must be wrong.* I bolted down the steps as Dale skidded to a halt, covering us both in a thick cloud of dust. Dale exploded out of the car.

"We have to leave, Paula. *Now.*" I followed him into the cabin as he breathlessly barked the words: "We have to leave in ten minutes. Can you do that?"

"What's happened? Is something wrong? Dale, you're scaring me."

"Honey, I just picked up a phone message from Dr. Cohen. It was her personally." Turning to face me, Dale continued. "She is going to be in San Diego, but only today, and is willing to meet with us. Can you believe that? She's going to meet with you . . . help you!"

I was stunned. "What? How did this happen?"

"We have to leave now. Right now. Please, Paula, trust me. Get everything into the car as fast as you can. I'll explain the details on the way, okay?"

For the next several minutes Dale and I tore through the cabin like a couple of human tornadoes, grabbing our belongings, picking up books, papers, videos—all the materials scattered throughout. I hurriedly checked the drawers and bathroom, throwing everything into my suitcase. As I stacked piles of our belongings at the front door, Dale grabbed them and headed to the car, tossing them haphazardly wherever they would fit. Within minutes, we were strapped in, tires spinning, engine screeching as we raced down the narrow winding road toward the highway.

Dale whipped the car around curves as if we were conducting trial runs for the Indy 500. I held my breath. Grabbing the door handle with one hand and holding onto the dashboard with the other, I tried to stay upright around a dozen big turns. The car swerved back and forth, slapping me against the door, then throwing me into the center console. My head was snapping back and forth like a palm tree in a hurricane. "Slow down, Dale. You've got to slow down." I was almost ready to give up my breakfast.

"I'm sorry, Paula. You're right. Sorry."

Dale slowed the car a bit and I finally breathed easier. "Okay, Dale. Tell me how you set up this meeting. I still can't believe you did it."

"You know the Bible says, 'You have not because you ask not.' Right?"

I slowly nodded in agreement. "Yes."

"Well, two days ago I tracked down Dr. Cohen's Phoenix phone number. I called and spoke to her assistant, requesting a meeting—anyplace, anytime. Of course, I offered to pay a sizable amount of money if the doctor would see us, but she doesn't see patients anymore. No exceptions.

"Anyway, I called again yesterday. I spoke to the same lady, begging her to ask Dr. Cohen to consider making an exception. I told her you were given three to six months to live unless you did all the conventional treatments: surgery, chemo, and radiation. But you were committed to following an alternative path, just as Dr. Cohen had done and just as she described on her videos. I told the assistant we were both pastors and you believed God led you to Dr. Cohen's information, but we had specific questions and really hoped we could speak with her face-to-face. I stressed the fact that I believe the Bible verse that says, 'A workman is worthy of his wages.' I told her we'd pay whatever reasonable fee she was accustomed to getting, or more if necessary. I hate to admit it, but I broke down during our conversation. I don't know what's wrong with me . . . I got pretty emotional. Anyway, I gave her our phone number and pleaded with her to ask Dr. Cohen to consider meeting with us. I let her know we could be in Phoenix with about eight hours' notice . . . or meet her anywhere she prefers."

"Oh my goodness, Dale. How wonderful of you. But I can't believe you didn't tell me."

"Well, Paula, it didn't seem likely it would happen. And I didn't think it was wise to get your hopes up knowing it would take a miracle to meet with her in person. Anyway, today when I picked up phone messages, there was a call from Dr. Cohen . . . *personally.* It was her, not her assistant, and she *is* willing to see us but it has to be today at two o'clock. She is flying in to San Diego for one day and can meet us at the corporate jet terminal at Lindbergh Field."

"Oh, Dale . . . I can't believe you were able to get us an appointment. Thank you."

"Well, praise the Lord. God is the One who opened these doors . . . that's for sure. Oh, by the way, we're going to rendezvous with Kara at the bottom of the hill. She really wants to come with us. That's partly why we had to leave so quickly. I called her from town just to let her know what had happened, but you know Kara. She's clamoring at any opportunity to be in the middle of whatever God is doing. You don't mind, do you?"

"Of course not." Our nineteen-year-old daughter, the younger of our two children, remained especially close even though she had moved out on her own several months earlier. This new battle with cancer had bonded us more tightly than ever. "It will be like a crash course for her to catch up with much of what we've learned. But we'll have to meet Kara and somehow still be at the airport in two and a half hours . . . how can we make it?"

I felt the car accelerate as my heart soared and my mind raced with a million questions I wanted to ask the doctor. "Where's my makeup? I have to fix myself up a bit." As I turned to find my cosmetic case in the backseat, my heart stopped. "Where's Wicket? Didn't you get him? Where's the dog?" My stomach lurched as panic set in.

Dale slammed on the brakes while yanking the car to the side of the road. "No. I thought you got him. Oh, my gosh!" In a heartbeat Dale shifted into low gear, flooring the accelerator while spinning the steering wheel 180 degrees. Within seconds our car was catapulted back up the winding mountain road while we both nervously scanned the shoulders for little Wicket.

As the cabin came into view, so did the dog. There he sat. Calmly and patiently waiting on the porch next to the chair where I had been sitting just minutes earlier. Racing up the steps, I grabbed him in one swoop, apologizing all the way back to the car. No sooner had I closed my door than we were a dragster once again, racing down the hill. *Maybe I won't have to deal with cancer after all. I might just die in a fiery car crash on the way to San Diego . . .*

———————————

Pacing back and forth, waiting for the "doc" to arrive, I was wearing a path in the plush carpet of the conference room. The three of us had made it to our destination with time to spare. I still couldn't believe Dale hadn't gotten a speeding ticket.

The moment we entered the corporate jet terminal, Dale arranged to use a private conference room. This was his territory. He had used these same facilities on several occasions while working with pilots and clients in the corporate jet transportation service we had owned and operated several years before.

Until this time, everything I had come to know about cancer was from doctors, patients, books, and videos. This meeting would be my first face-to-face encounter with a live person who had used an alternative approach to fight cancer—and had won. Not only that, but she was a highly experienced and credentialed medical doctor. That seemed like an oxymoron.

"Sit down, Paula. You're making me nervous." Dale sat at the large table, arranging his legal pad and pen.

I couldn't sit. My palms were sweaty. I had trouble swallowing. "I'll sit when she gets here. I'm trying to watch for her car so she knows where we are." I pulled the louvers of the floor-length vertical blinds aside, peering into the parking lot.

Dale sighed. "Honey, she'll likely be in a taxi or a vehicle with airport terminal markings."

"I think she just pulled up! Oh, my gosh. This is *exciting.*" My heart was pounding.

Dr. Cohen looked twenty years younger than her age, which she had revealed on the videos. The vibrancy she exuded spoke volumes about her health and fitness. I could scarcely believe this was the woman I had seen on the TV screen. But it had to be. *She looks exactly like the person in the videos, but how could it be? So much time has passed . . . doesn't she age?*

Dale rose to sneak a look through the blinds. "Good grief, she looks young enough to be my little sister."

When I walked outside to greet her, I noticed there were no flaws in her skin. She looked to be in perfect health. For a woman who had been so sick to look so youthfully vibrant said a lot to me about her credibility. "Hi, I'm Paula. Thanks for meeting with us. We're in here." I directed her into the conference room and introduced her to Dale and Kara.

She smiled warmly while shaking hands. "As I told you on the phone, I don't usually meet with people. But Dale, you convinced me that you two were not only desperate but also very serious about taking the right kind of action. And I felt somehow that God is in this, so I made an exception."

Dale spoke up. "Paula and I believe God led us to you, so I had to make every effort to get us together. I'm so grateful you were willing to meet. Thank you so very much." Matter-of-factly, Dale slid the check he had prepared across the table toward her. "Please use this to get us started. And somehow, I'll get more later. You have my word . . ."

Dr. Cohen interrupted. "I'm not doing this for money, Dale." She handed the check back. "I go as I feel directed by the Lord. It's my pleasure to be here. I'm here to help."

The doctor took a seat at the oval cherrywood table opposite me, with Dale seated at one end and Kara at the other. I noticed that she carried a bright blue bottle of drinking water, which she placed on the table next to her.

With a warm smile, Dr. Cohen glanced around the table. "It's so nice to meet all of you." The pleasantries over, Dr. Cohen got right to the point of our meeting. "Paula, Dale told me on the phone that you've been diagnosed with breast cancer and have been given three to six months unless you follow conventional procedures." The doctor studied my face, her eyes fixed on mine. "Is that your situation, Paula?"

"Yes, that pretty much covers it." I pushed the pathology report and my medical records across the table. I wanted her professional input. It was an unexpected relief to be speaking to a woman who empathized with what I was feeling—she had walked the road I was now traveling. And even though she was

157

a highly respected medical doctor, I knew she had reversed her cancer with the new direction Dale and I were pursuing.

She scanned through my medical paperwork in silence. I wondered what she was thinking. I didn't have long to wait.

Dr. Cohen lifted her gaze and locked her eyes on mine. Her next words were few—but intense. "Paula . . . your situation is extremely serious. You're a *very, very* sick woman."

CHAPTER 15

The Doctor Is In

⌒

Dr. Cohen's evaluation of how sick I was caught me off guard—shocked me into reality. I finally had to admit to myself that I *was* indeed very sick. That if I didn't do the right things—*now*—I was in imminent danger of dying of cancer. And there are no "do-overs" with dying. Dr. Cohen's pronouncement was a real wake-up call. Her message came crashing through loud and clear, but there was something else happening too.

Out of the corner of my eye, I noticed Kara trembling in her chair and struggling to hold back her tears—unsuccessfully. Tenderhearted Kara was having her own reaction to Dr. Cohen's ominous words. Seeing her tears stopped me in my tracks. *She's afraid I might die. And if I don't find more answers quickly, I just might.*

For the first time, the cancer threat to my life became glaringly real. It was no longer out "there" somewhere. It was now close and personal. But as I looked at Kara and Dale and thought about our son, new electrifying conviction charged through me. *I will not die of cancer. I will get well. I will do whatever I have to do. I will take immediate and extreme action. I will do anything and everything to live. I owe it to Kara. I owe it to Dale and Eric and the rest of my family. I also owe it to myself. But most of all, I owe it to the God who loves me and is showing me my way of escape.*

I straightened my back and turned toward the doctor. "I choose life, Dr. Cohen. I am willing to do *everything* needed." I looked at Kara and Dale: "I am going to live. I promise you!"

My eyes fell again on Dr. Cohen and I chuckled. "Gosh, in many ways it's easier to die than to do what it takes to live. But Doc, you show me what to do for my body, and I'll do whatever is needed to live. I know how to walk in faith and how to keep my spirit strong. I understand the need for the right heart-talk, the right attitude and thoughts in the soulish realm. I'm not where I need to be yet, but I've been there in the past and I do know what to do to get there again. But what I haven't known before is about my body. Between what Dale and I have been discovering and what you're teaching us, I will learn whatever is necessary and then *do* all that is required."

I feel good! Exhilarated! I had staked a claim to my new future. Battle lines had been drawn. I was going on the offensive, taking a stand. But these weren't just feelings. I was filled with resolve. *I will seek out the enemy—and win this war.*

Kara wiped the tears from her eyes while flashing me a tentative smile. I think it helped her to hear my affirmation. I glanced over at Dale, expecting an emotional pat on the back for my positive stand. But he was slumped over the table, his face in both hands as he choked out the words, "I'm sorry, you guys."

I stared, trying to assimilate what this meant. After a brief pause, he looked up with tear-filled eyes. "I know there's no crying in baseball."

We all laughed.

Ever since I had been diagnosed, Dale had been unflinching

in holding fear at bay with his confidence and encouragement. He had faithfully been the strength of our family—always positive, always cheering me on. But I was now taking over. He had primed the pump but now I was in gear . . . really, for the first time since learning I had cancer. Deep down I knew that's how it had to be. No one else could face this enemy for me. This was a battle I had to fight, a war I had to win.

Dr. Cohen settled back in her chair and smiled. "It's great to hear that, Paula. I'm really pleased, for your sakes." She took a sip from her water bottle. "It is so important for patients to be that determined to get better—but they rarely are. It's also unusual for people to challenge conventional medical treatments." Dr. Cohen looked my direction. "Paula, your approach, along with your commitment, will most certainly save your life.

"Okay, tell me what you both know so far. Paula, you mentioned that you feel God is revealing a Body-Soul-Spirit approach for your healing. Before I share with you about the body, could you first briefly tell me about the spirit and soul parts of your approach so I can understand your perspective of these vitally important areas?"

"Of course. Well, the spirit is the most important in my opinion. Death is inevitable, so we all need to confront life-after-death. But dealing with cancer really brings that reality home. God has been a vital part of our lives ever since Dale and I met. We understand how important it is for the Bible to be the highest authority in our spiritual growth and a guiding influence in our lives. We've tried diligently to *live* by His Word, not just know it intellectually.

"With God as my foundation and His Word as my plumb line, I can find His will in any situation. First, and most importantly, I know that when I die, I will go to heaven. But since the Bible tells me God wants me healed, when I learned I had cancer, I asked Him to heal me and lead me into truth."

Dr. Cohen nodded. "Those are two critically important parts of any plan. What else?"

"By clinging to God's Word, I have more peace, less stress, and more hope and faith in my daily life."

Dale added, "But we also know this world is a battlefield in many ways. We know—beyond any doubt—that God is a healing God. His will is to heal and answer prayer. We are confident God's will is to heal Paula of cancer because the Bible tells us in Psalms 103:3 that God heals all our diseases. What we didn't know was *how* God would do that, but now Paula believes that this Body-Soul-Spirit approach is her way of escape. And I agree. It incorporates biblical principles with natural laws of health. It also just makes sense to me."

"Okay, I agree, but now tell me about the 'soul' part of your plan."

"I am aware that for me to get well and stay well, I must eliminate things like worry, resentment,

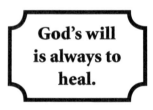

God's will is always to heal.

anger, and unforgiveness from my life. These things affect both my spirit and my soul. If I don't deal with them, they can manifest in my physical body in negative ways."

"You are so right, Paula. I have had many patients who are angry with someone and harbor resentment or unforgiveness. Not only do these emotions *cause* sickness and disease because of the stresses they put on the body, but they also make it difficult to get well. When patients refuse to let go, the bitterness continues to poison their body with toxic stress hormones that weaken the immune system more and more."

I nodded. "Now I understand that, Doc. I'm sure that's why God tells us to always forgive others and not to be angry. He knows what those emotions do to our body. My mind, will, and emotions make up the soul part of me and are a huge area of concern in my quest for health. I realize that my spirit, soul, and body are all connected and each part affects the others. It's automatic . . . it's the way we're created. Without God's help in the area of the soul, I don't know how to eliminate these negative thoughts and emotions effectively and permanently."

The doc asked, "Paula, are you angry at God for this cancer?"

"No way. And I never was angry. At first, I did ask 'why.' But God didn't send this to me. I'm aware that He doesn't work that way. I may have unknowingly violated the natural way He designed me to live and function, but now I'm ready to make all the changes necessary to get well. Besides, how could I blame Him or think He caused it and then ask Him to heal me? That wouldn't make any sense. Doc, you should know that Dale and I have diligently prayed for God to heal me of cancer. I asked the elders of our church to pray and lay hands on me too, according to Scripture. I was even anointed with oil. I did everything the Bible told me to do." I paused. "And I've seen miracles take place. I believe in them and know God can do that at any time. But I also believe that I need to continue searching for the truth about what I can do to work in agreement with Him for my healing."

The doctor leaned toward me. "Paula, if you find the truth . . . will you believe it?"

I chuckled. "I have to admit, it's been a challenge to believe things so contrary to what I've been taught all my life. But these new discoveries ring true according to God's Word *and* in my heart. I believe God has answered my prayers by leading me to the truth. So, yes. I've made the decision to believe it."

"Good." Dr. Cohen smiled. "This information *is* in stark contradiction to what the public has been taught. But isn't it freeing when you embrace truth?"

Dale jumped in. "It really is! And suddenly other things make sense. It's like turning on a light that makes all the objects in the room visible so I can understand what they are and how to use or avoid them."

"Exactly. Well said, Dale. I'm pleased to hear all this. You know, I see people all the time who change their diet—are diligent about their body—yet die of cancer. I now believe that what you two call the Body-Soul-Spirit approach to overcoming sickness and disease, in particular cancer, is vital because it addresses the whole person. And the best results are when all parts are healed, not just one part. I'm glad for your sakes you have these aspects firmly intact."

Dale spoke again. "Doc, I must admit we are still struggling with some of our thoughts—the mind part of the soul. We know the Bible says that 'as a man thinks in his heart, so is he.'[37] But we know that Paula must not think of herself as a cancer victim."

"That's right," I added. "I can't think of myself as a person with cancer who's trying to get well. On the contrary, I have to think of myself as already healed, with leftover symptoms that will eventually leave my body. I've prayed with faith and asked God to heal me and lead me into truth. Now I must act on His Word and live out that belief—not in foolish ignorance but in wise perseverance. I'm a healed person. Give me just a few more days. I'll get my faith fully in gear."

"Oh, that sounds great. That's a bull's-eye. You have the spirit and soul parts of healing in place. Well done. Now, let's focus on the body. What do you know so far?"

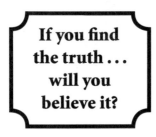

If you find the truth . . . will you believe it?

Dr. Cohen listened attentively as I recounted the highlights of the information we had recently learned about the body from the books and other materials in our "life" pile, culminating with her information from the videotapes.

"The information about the body and how it deals with

cancer is new to us," I explained, "but what we've learned makes a lot of sense."

Dr. Cohen nodded. "You're on the right track. Your understanding that standard medical treatments for cancer are both dangerous and destructive is vital. You have to pull out the weeds before you plant the flowers. It's the same if you're going to start any natural method of healing. You have to avoid or stop the damaging treatments so your body can respond to the natural process.

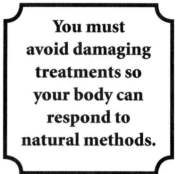

"Look, you two are quite different from most people I come across. You seem to have the spiritual part of healing in place already. You also seem to understand what is needed in your mind and attitude. You're doing great in those areas. Many people I hear from think that getting well is all about diet. Diet is important, true, but it's only a part of what it takes to get well. As I said, I've seen many people strictly follow a natural diet and die anyway. It's more than just diet. Please don't forget that.

"Okay, it seems clear that I can help you most in the area of the body, so that's what I'll focus on. Agreed?"

Dale and I nodded.

"We agree, doctor," I affirmed. "That sounds like the best use of your time."

"May I ask one question?" Kara lifted her hand just enough to get everyone's attention. "Dr. Cohen, are you saying that you really believe the approach my mom's doctor recommended—surgery, chemo, and radiation—is *not* the way to go?"

Alternative methods were still new to Kara. We hadn't been able to share the details of our Body-Soul-Spirit approach with her yet. It had taken Dale and me well over a week of intensive research to discover that there are natural ways to reverse cancer and other diseases, and Kara was trying to catch up. I was grateful she was hearing these truths from a medical doctor who was also a woman completely cured of terminal cancer. It would help give her the confidence that this approach would work for me too.

Dr. Cohen took the time to explain. "That's right, Kara. I was diagnosed with advanced terminal cancer. But as a medical doctor, I knew that standard treatment would *not* save my life. I knew if I went to the hospital and followed normal medical protocol for cancer, it would kill me. Instead, I diligently searched every alternative method available until I found my way through the maze. Eventually, I reversed my cancer with a godly and natural alternative approach. I got well without radiation or chemotherapy. And your mom can do the same."

Kara still looked skeptical. "I don't mean any disrespect, Dr. Cohen, but are you actually saying that Mom should not have *any* chemo or radiation treatments?"

The doc shook her head emphatically. "Do you really think chemotherapy can cure cancer? It's a powerful, lethal drug. Chemotherapy kills both good and bad cells that are fast growing. Tumors are fast growing, yes. But so are the cells of the immune system—and that is the *only* system that actually fights cancer. But there's much more. Drugs can't cure disease. Chemotherapy is a drug—it *cannot* cure cancer. At best, drugs suppress symptoms. Let me repeat that. Drugs can't cure cancer. And all drugs have side effects that often cause added distress in our bodies.

> **Chemotherapy is a drug. Drugs don't cure cancer. Drugs only treat symptoms.**

"Let's also talk about radiation. Radiation can't cure cancer either. Radiation only deals with the symptoms of cancer—the tumor, not the cause. And radiation does immense damage to healthy cells too. Oh, did I mention that both chemotherapy and radiation do serious damage to the immune system? And they can also *cause* cancer!

"Listen, the medical system is broken. It's completely upside down. When it comes to disease, we doctors are trained only to treat symptoms. Doctors don't deal with root causes. That's how the medical system works. And when it comes to cancer, doctors are taught only to cut, poison, or burn out tumors—with surgery, chemotherapy, or radiation. But none of these methods treat the cause of cancer at all—they only deal with the tumors. Yet tumors are *not* the cancer. Tumors are the *symptoms* of cancer. The 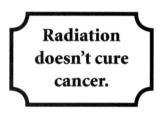 patient sometimes shows temporary signs of improvement from chemotherapy and radiation. However, these treatments actually make the cancer worse, not better. And they don't deal with the reason cancer developed to begin with."

Dale looked at Dr. Cohen. "That's exactly what we've been learning. And it's shocking. No one in the medical industry is addressing the *cause* of the cancer. We've researched enough already to understand that the treatments the doctors recommend for Paula don't address why she *has* cancer. And if she got cancer once, why wouldn't she get it again? I mean, hello-o."

"Precisely. And that's a great question, Dale. Paula got cancer because her immune system quit functioning properly. It happened to her gradually, weakening more and more, one day at a time, until finally she reached a tipping point. It's really quite logical. As you've already learned, everyone has cancer cells in their body, even babies. The problem begins when our healthy cells cannot destroy the damaged cancer cells fast enough.

"Remember, cancer results from a broken-down immune

LIFE, CANCER AND GOD

system. If your body is undernourished or dehydrated . . . or you deal poorly with stress . . . your immune system weakens. And it may become too weak to effectively handle the countless toxins your normal daily life and diet produce. Cancer is the result of a suppressed immune system—plain and simple. You need to add the nutrients and water your body needs, but you also have to stop taking in toxins from stress and things like smoking, prescription medicine, processed foods, preservatives and additives, pesticides, chemicals, and similar harmful things."

I watched Kara. *How much of this is she absorbing?* Her jaw had dropped and her eyes were riveted on the doctor's face as she spoke. *This is working. Kara is beginning to catch up.* I breathed a sigh of relief.

Kara commented, "Dr. Cohen, you mentioned that undernourishment can cause cancer. I don't understand that. It seems odd to me because there's so much cancer in this country yet people mostly get enough food. I mean, lots of people who have cancer are even overweight."

"Okay, Kara. You're right. But how much someone eats has nothing to do with nutrition. People in our country are getting plenty of calories—that's for sure. That's not the problem. I'm talking about nutrients—vitamins, minerals, and enzymes. And not from supplements but in natural forms—from real foods. It's about getting enough of the *right* nutrients into our system to nourish our cells and strengthen our immune system. That only happens with the right kinds of food—and most people eat the wrong foods. Therefore, we have a cancer epidemic. Does that make sense?"

> **Cancer is the result of a suppressed immune system— plain and simple.**

"Oh . . . I think I get it." Kara settled back in her chair. I could see the wheels turning. "So you're saying we have either so many damaged cells caused by stress or toxins that our good cells can't keep up . . . or our good cells are so weak from a lack of nutrition and hydration that they can't fight even a normal number of damaged cells."

"That's essentially correct," Dr. Cohen replied. "And then when the cancer cells start multiplying in one area unchecked, they form a tumor. A tumor tells you that your body is in critical danger. It usually takes years for a tumor to grow large enough to detect, which means your immune system has been weakened for a long time. When cancer is discovered, it's not just your breast or prostate or lung that's having a problem. Cancer is a systemic disease. If you have cancer anywhere, it means your entire system is compromised."

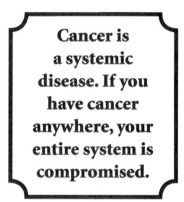

Cancer is a systemic disease. If you have cancer anywhere, your entire system is compromised.

I am so grateful Kara is hearing such a credible source share this revolutionary information firsthand.

Knowing cancer had cut a path through my side of the family aroused questions from Kara about heredity. "Dr. Cohen, how high is my risk for getting cancer? My grandmother had it. Several aunts, my grandpa, and now my mom. Is it a sure thing that I'll get cancer someday too? My doctor says I'm high risk."

The doctor smiled politely. "Oh, Kara, let me explain. Contrary to what you've undoubtedly heard and read, with rare exceptions, cancer is *not* hereditary. Cancer is passed down through families all right, but not through the genes. Now I'm aware that your doctor asks many questions about the diseases of your family. But doctors are trained incorrectly. Let me make myself clear. With only minor exceptions, cancer is passed down by *training* the child how to eat, drink, think, and how to cope with stress. Cancer is not handed down by the genes."

Kara leaned back in her chair. "Whew! That's a relief." Then after a moment's pause, "But, really?"

"Yes, really. You see, cancer is passed down by habit patterns, behavioral models in the home. I mean, mom eats poorly, doesn't handle stress well, has unresolved emotional issues, loads herself with toxins daily, and then one day, bam, she's diagnosed with cancer. And it doesn't matter if it's brain cancer, breast cancer, lung cancer, cancer of the blood, or any other kind. Cancer is cancer. Well, mom taught her daughter how to live this way. So daughter eats poorly, doesn't handle stress well, has unresolved emotional issues, loads herself with toxins, and then one day—wouldn't you know it—*she's* diagnosed with cancer too." Dr. Cohen frowned. "The medical industry calls this *genetically induced*. That's not even logical. Think of it this way, Kara. Cancer is not passed down through the genes. Cancer-producing habits are passed down through *lifestyle.*

"Listen, all of you. Many studies have been done that draw on the lives of adopted children as compared with natural-born children to the same parents. These studies are conclusive. Cancer is *not* a genetic disease. It is scarcely hereditary. So, Kara, don't worry about getting cancer just because your mom and grandmother and other family members have had it. But don't take the threat lightly either. Learn all you can now. And Kara, listen carefully, honey. Make necessary lifestyle changes

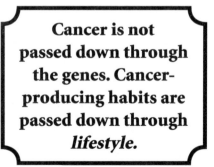

Cancer is not passed down through the genes. Cancer-producing habits are passed down through *lifestyle.*

starting now. Learn how to live in a way that you will never, ever develop cancer. You *can* prevent this disease. You don't have to get cancer. Ever. Not only that, but if you live in a way that prevents cancer, you'll also be avoiding most other diseases at the same time.

"As I've mentioned, I am fully retired from practicing medicine. I almost never meet patients like this anymore. So, Kara, listen and learn." The doctor pointed to Dale and me, both taking notes.

Kara smiled and pulled out pen and paper. "Good idea, Doc. Why didn't you think of that sooner?"

The doctor's mouth dropped open.

Dale and I just shook our heads.

CHAPTER 16

Cause and Effect

⟿

*M*y head was swimming. Every answer brought up more questions. I had never learned so much so fast, but still had no answers to one particular question that had been needling me for some time. "Dr. Cohen, could you please explain why people get cancer more than once?"

"It's actually quite common. If the people with cancer don't change anything at the root level to increase their system's ability to eliminate the damaged cells, then they are sitting ducks to have a new tumor form somewhere in their body. In addition, if they had chemotherapy, radiation, or both, they have further devastated their immune system—which, as I've said, is the *only* system in the body that actually fights cancer. The treatments doctors routinely prescribe all but obliterate the very system the patient needs most.

"Many things can damage and deplete a person's immune system, but there's only one way to fix it: The immune system must be rebuilt and strengthened naturally. This isn't a quick fix, and there are no shortcuts. But cancer can be reversed when the patient is dedicated to making the changes needed to bring his or her system back to health. Paula, you can do this with certainty of success. And don't worry about cancer returning. I've been cancer free for over a decade—without radiation or chemo. In fact, I've never been healthier."

I responded, "Well, it certainly shows."

She smiled. "Thank God."

Dr. Cohen was sharing many of the same truths Dale and I had discovered during our research in the mountains. God was leading me in the same way He had led her. I was both stunned and excited. The doc was providing powerful confirmation to our newly discovered Body-Soul-Spirit approach.

Kara, who had been squirming in her chair for a couple of minutes, spat out a question. "Dr. Cohen, why isn't Mom's doctor explaining any of this? It's hard to believe that the doctors and hospitals don't know this stuff and don't do what's really needed to help cancer patients get well. I've met Dr. Anderson and he seems like a great doctor. He's a nice man and I like him."

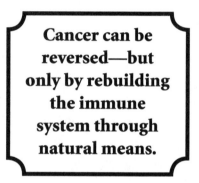

Cancer can be reversed—but only by rebuilding the immune system through natural means.

The doc's eyes darted from Kara's to Dale's to mine, where they locked in place. "Paula, has your doctor mentioned any treatments besides surgery, chemo, and radiation?"

"No, he has not. Dale asked if there was anything I could do while waiting for the next surgery, but the doctor said, no, nothing. He told me I just have to wait for the chemo and radiation to do their job."

Dr. Cohen rolled her eyes and shook her head. Her voice rose slightly, punctuating her terse response. "See? That's what I'm talking about. There's a protocol for cancer in place that doctors cannot violate without huge liability and personal cost. If a patient is given any treatment outside the party line and the patient dies, the doctor can be considered liable. Plus, the medical industry will crucify any doctor who violates protocol, so they stay with the herd. They place protection of their careers over protection of their patients. If you want to be a successful doctor in this world's system, you do what you're trained to do—what's expected of you.

"Now I understand that what I'm saying is difficult to believe because it's a different way of looking at the medical community. But cancer is big business and brings in hundreds of billions of dollars every year. The doctors are just the middlemen, the salespeople for the drug companies, the bridge between the public and the powers that control this mega machine. And no one wants to rock this colossal money boat."

While still looking down, quickly scribbling notes, I responded, "Wow. What you are teaching us is powerful information. You're also confirming Dale's research. On one hand, this *is* difficult to accept." I lifted my eyes and gazed at Dr. Cohen. "On the other hand, with this new perspective, so many things I didn't understand before now make complete sense."

"I sympathize with your shock, Paula, but it doesn't change what's true. People keep burying their heads. Very few question the system. Patients are dying in unbelievable numbers—in what I consider a medical holocaust. But you must remember something. Countless patients are reversing disease amid all this fraudulent behavior. Many are finding alternative approaches—and getting well, usually *after* the doctors have told them nothing more can be done. The medical system gives them all it has to give, then throws them out to die. That's when some who don't give up find an effective alternative approach. Thousands and thousands have reversed the disease. Unfortunately, most patients die before finding the truth because most never look for it. And others look, but they look in the wrong places."

I need a solid handle on my course of action. Now's my chance to get her input. "Dr. Cohen, with the many alternative methods used to reverse cancer, which ones do you find most helpful?"

The doctor laughed aloud. "Oh, my goodness. There were nearly a hundred different alternative approaches when I was searching. I evaluated all I could find and then tried the most promising ones. Most did not work for me. I mean so many people are offering quick fixes, trying to pull a rabbit out of a hat. It's a jungle out there, and people who have cancer are so desperate they'll consider anything that promises a cure. Then there are some programs so close to God's design that you can find many golden nuggets of truth.

"But let me caution you," she continued, turning serious. "Any medical doctor—I'm talking about a licensed and experienced medical professional—who turns to alternative medicine will be crucified by their peers and by the medical industry. There are big dollars available to protect the status quo. The big pharmaceutical companies, the American Medical Association, and the National Cancer Institute work diligently to make examples of the medical professionals who break rank. They can't afford for others to follow so they handle these people one way—by attacking their reputations and destroying their credibility. So if any of the alternative programs you find are championed by a former physician or medical professional, you have to sift through and ignore much of the slander written about that person. Sometimes there's even more than slander—there are lawsuits, personal persecution, and outright lies. It's wise to evaluate the program more than the person who's leading it."

Dale's antennae went up. "Yeah, we read about Dr. Max

Gerson. He was discredited, slandered, and persecuted. Remember, Paula?"

I nodded.

Dr. Cohen responded. "Many believe he was also murdered. Killed for his tremendous success in reversing cancer. It seems that the more successful people are in cancer reversal or disease prevention, the more persecution they experience."

Throwing up my hands, I had to speak. "It's unbelievable that someone would actually be murdered to stop such life-giving news."

There was silence for a few moments. Then Dale commented, "It's a lot like the prophets of the Bible. In essence, they were killed for speaking the truth—the truth that came from God for the people. Most people don't really want the truth. They want only what they want. Seldom do they seek the *complete* truth. But what we're discussing in this room is the truth. And I believe these are truths God wants His people to know about."

A knock on the door interrupted our conversation. The door slowly opened just enough to allow the receptionist to squeeze her head through. "Sorry for the intrusion, but, Dr. Cohen? You have a call at the front desk."

"Oh, thank you. I'll be right there." Turning to me, she explained, "I've been expecting this call and I really need to take it. Can we have a break for . . . oh, let's say about fifteen or twenty minutes?"

"Of course, no problem," I replied. "We'll be waiting for you back here. Take whatever time you need, and please know that we appreciate your help so very much."

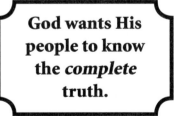

God wants His people to know the *complete* truth.

It felt good to stand and stretch. Glancing at my watch, I could hardly believe we had been talking for over an hour. I turned toward Dale. "Why don't I call the house for messages while we have some time?"

"Sure," he smiled. "That's a good idea. There are a lot of them, so brace yourself—I didn't erase any. Kara and I will take a little walk. I'd like to show her the Learjet 35 parked on the tarmac. She doesn't seem to remember the days I flew all over the world in them. We even took her on many of our flights, but she was pretty young. We'll meet you back here in a few minutes."

I headed toward the pilots' lounge to make my call. As expected, the answering machine was full. *Yep, that's part of why we left for the mountains.* I waded through the calls—most from well-wishers and friends just checking to see how I was doing. Writing down the names and numbers, I was grateful for my loved ones. *I'm ready to communicate with them again.*

Then I heard a message left only an hour before our meeting began. It was a voice in distress—Jada's voice, my dear friend from the cancer club.

"Hi, Paula. This is Jada." Her voice quivered. "I got some bad news. I thought maybe you and I could pray together. The doctor just found cancer in my lungs and lower spine." Her voice broke. "The cancer has spread and it's bad. I don't know what to do." After remaining silent for a moment, Jada finished her message through smothered sobs. "I'm getting worse, Paula. Please call me when you can. I'd really like to talk to you . . . and pray together. Love you. Bye." Her voice sounded strained and small.

The hope that had been building within me now dimmed. A fog of fear and confusion threatened to envelop me. *How can Jada be worse? A lot worse.* My heart sank. She had become such a wonderful friend. In the brief time since we'd met, we had spoken on the phone often, praying and building our faith together. I hadn't considered that things would get worse for her. Dale and I had spent time with Jada and her daughter just before taking our trip to the mountains. She had been optimistic and hopeful, doing everything she could to get better. At least everything Dr. Anderson had recommended.

In one blinding instant, Jada's words collided with my new understanding. *I do know. I know exactly why Jada's cancer has spread. But I don't want to believe this is happening to such a wonderful person and dear friend.* I thought of all I'd learned since we'd arrived in the mountains. *How can such a special person like Jada become progressively worse and maybe even die of cancer when there is such an abundance of truth available?*

Needing to talk to someone who was thinking clearly, I hurried out of the pilots' lounge, looking for Dale. Spotting him and Kara outside next to a sleek twin-engine jet, I scurried in their direction.

Dale took one look at my face and started toward me. "What's wrong, Paula?"

Tears started to fall. Wrapping my arms around his waist, I buried my face in his chest as my words poured out. "Jada called. She's much worse. The cancer has spread to her lungs and spine. It's real bad, Dale. Jada is in serious trouble." My tears turned into sobs.

The threat of the deadly disease Jada and I were carrying in our bodies came rushing back with a vengeance. *Am I really finding the way to be healed of cancer—my way of escape? Or am I fooling myself?* A knot tightened in my stomach. My chest constricted. "We can't lose Jada, Dale. We're learning so many things that can help her. We can't lose our precious friend . . . not now. We're finally discovering the truth about cancer. It's not too late—is it?"

CHAPTER 17

Reversing Cancer Naturally

～

Lord, I'm so concerned about Jada, I can't even think! There is so much I want to tell her about what I'm discovering. Now more than ever, she needs this Body-Soul-Spirit information. As soon as this meeting is over, I'll go see her and share these lifesaving truths about reversing cancer.

Directing my focus back to our meeting, I wanted to listen to everything Dr. Cohen was saying. I needed to learn as much as possible—for myself, for Jada, and for the others in my cancer club. For all I knew, I'd never have this face-to-face opportunity again.

The doc was back in high gear. "Paula, Dale, Kara, there are laws that govern health. These laws are always at work, whether we know about them or not. If we violate them, we end up with sickness, disease, and premature death."

Kara blurted out a question. "But everyone has to die of something. We can't all live forever, right?"

Dr. Cohen smiled. "You're right, Kara. We can't live forever in these natural bodies, but we *can* live disease free until we die. Some people live to an old age in a healthy body and finally go to sleep and never wake up. Why can't we all do that? Why can't we just go to bed and die of old age when our time is up? I believe we can."

Dale spoke up. "That's exactly how my grandmother and grandfather died."

I nodded. "It's true. They just went to sleep. Neither one had any sickness or disease. They still lived in their own home. Grandma sensed her time was near and over the course of a couple of days, the entire family had the opportunity to go to the house and say good-bye. She was ninety-six when she went to sleep peacefully and woke up in heaven. It was a wonderful example of how God designed us to leave this world."

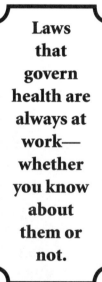

Laws that govern health are always at work—whether you know about them or not.

The doc responded. "That is rare these days, and it's refreshing to hear their story."

"Oh, and it's completely accurate," Dale confirmed. "I was with them almost daily during that time. And a few months later Grandpa died at age ninety-six as well—from missing his wife more than anything else."

Wanting to know more about alternative options, I asked, "Why don't we ever hear about the people who have been cured with a natural approach?"

"That's easy to explain. The big pharmaceutical and medical companies that make billions on the cancer business also spend millions on undermining the claims of alternative medicine. They work aggressively and spend many dollars labeling it 'quackery' and worse. There is a massive campaign to keep people moving through the conventional medical system."

Though I remembered reading similar claims in several of the books from our "life" pile, it helped to hear it again from a credible source like Dr. Cohen. "This is an entirely new way to think. It changes everything I've always believed about doctors and medicine."

"I understand that this way of looking at the medical industry is contrary to how the public is trained," the doctor replied. "But now you know. You can stick your head back down in the sand and stay in denial if you want to—to your own detriment. Or you can question what is happening and look at the information and statistics that are available and accept the truth. The medical system is broken. Standard cancer treatment doesn't work. There *is* a better way."

I could see the pain in the doc's face as she spoke. This was a raw nerve.

"It cost me my career when I realized the truth," she continued. "I had a great lifestyle with many accolades from colleagues, neighbors, friends, and family. I had prestige and money. Though I had worked extremely hard for years to develop my practice, when I learned what I'm telling you now, I could no longer in good conscience continue to practice medicine according to the status quo. To do so would require me to lie to my patients much of the time. To walk away from my career . . . wow, that wasn't easy. But when I got breast cancer, I knew there had to be a better way than the treatments the medical system offered."

"What did you do? What happened after that?" I asked.

"To begin with, I turned to God—for the first time in my life. I asked Him to forgive me of my sins and invited Jesus into my heart. Then I asked for His help in getting well and started looking into alternative treatments. I investigated many options and tried several. Eventually I came up with a combination of a couple of different treatments that lined up with God's Word and made sense to me as a doctor.

"Unfortunately, I got worse before I got better. In fact, I got so ill my family insisted on taking me to a hospital. But I knew that would be deadly so I refused to go. Well, it took months for my body to finally respond, but eventually the tumor began to shrink. Little by little, day by day, I continued to improve. The healthier I became, the more I realized I could never practice traditional medicine again. Turning to God and sticking to a natural health plan saved my life. I had learned truth, and once I did, I was accountable before God for what I knew. The truth cost me my career—but it also saved my life."

Dale responded, "Doc, you don't know this, but before sensing the call of God to become a minister, I was an airline pilot and a jet flight instructor and examiner with decades of training and experience. So I think I understand the dedication and effort it took to achieve your position. I hope you aren't offended by my saying I don't automatically respect doctors. People are often wowed by physicians, but I'm not. I am moved by people who put integrity, honesty, and the care of others ahead of their careers and personal gain." Dale's eyes became misty and his voice cracked. "You're a rare find, Doc. You've placed God first in your life. You've chosen truth over your career and the comforts of this world. To me, your life shines like a polished diamond. I can't begin to express how much respect I have for you."

"Thank you, Dale. I appreciate that. You know, sometimes the hardest part of being a conventionally trained doctor is that we need to 'unlearn' a tremendous amount of information before we are open to accepting the truth."

I jumped in, the doc's words hitting a chord. "That's the way most people are too. We've all been conditioned to think a certain way—about doctors and the medical system. It's difficult to be open to a new way of thinking about cancer without understanding what's wrong with what we already believe."

The doctor stood and walked over to a large white board

affixed to one of the walls of the conference room. "Let me explain the real truth about cancer in general terms. First, the various cancers are not really different from one another. We give them different names based on where they are discovered in the body, but every cancer is basically the same as every other cancer. And the way to reverse any of them is the same— whether it's lung, brain, liver, breast, prostate, or blood cancer. Let me clarify." Selecting a blue marker, she turned and wrote on the board in large capital letters, CANCER IS CANCER. Turning back to the three of us, she continued. "Contrary to what doctors would have you believe, all cancer is caused by the same thing and all cancers are reversed in the same way. You got that? And to reverse cancer—any kind of cancer—one must . . ." She wrote these words: Rebuild and strengthen the immune system. "It's not really rocket science, kiddos."

Dale responded, "We're sold, Dr. Cohen." Laughing, he added, "But I like rocket science."

She smiled. "I'll keep that in mind, Dale. Now here's a question: What causes cancer? Answer: Cancer is the result of a repressed immune system. So play along with me now. Question: How can one reverse cancer? Answer: By rebuilding and strengthening one's immune system. That's basic Cancer 101. You see, if the immune system is working properly, it is not possible for cancer to develop."

She turned and wrote on the board again. Cancer = weak immune system. "So since you have cancer, Paula, and you could not have gotten cancer if your immune system had been working normally, then building up your God-given immune system is the only way to cure your cancer, isn't it? It's the way to cure most any disease."

Kara asked, "Just what exactly is the immune system?"

> If your immune system is working properly, it is not possible for you to get cancer.

The doctor turned back to the board and began writing. *Lymphoid.* "The immune system is a complex but vital network of cells and organs that protects the body against infection, bacteria, viruses, and fungi." She drew the outline of a human body and filled it with lines and small ovals representing the veins and lymph system that run throughout the entire body.

"A quick answer, Kara, is that blood vessels and lymphatic vessels make up lymphoid organs. The appendix, adenoids, bone marrow, lymph nodes, and a thing called Peyer's patches—tissues of the small intestine—all make up lymphoid organs. They affect growth, development, and the release of lymphocytes, infection-fighting white blood cells. There's more, but these are the basics. You see, it involves multiple organs and systems, so that's why it's called the immune *system.* All these parts work in harmony to protect the body. Does that answer your question well enough?"

"Sure." Kara nodded. "This is like going back to biology class."

"My thoughts exactly," I added. "But it sure helps me understand why my immune system is so important. It's all through my body."

Still standing, Dr. Cohen continued. "You have to come to grips with the cancer in your body and ask yourself how you got it. What or who caused the cancer? Was it a foreign invader? This is what health professionals would like you to believe. But no, it wasn't something foreign. In fact, *you* caused your own cancer. Just as I caused mine. Understanding this principle was a real eye-opener for me. I had to come to grips with that truth to get well. Paula, you gave yourself cancer. I don't mean to sound harsh, but the truth sometimes comes across that way at first. Whether knowingly or unknowingly, you caused cancer in your body. Do you want to know why that's good news?"

"I sure do. It doesn't sound like good news."

"Well, since you caused it, you can reverse it. It's about cause and effect. You are *not* the victim here, Paula. You didn't just randomly get invaded with this disease. Instead, you brought this on yourself. The good news is you can reverse it yourself."

"And I'm determined to do just that."

"It's really frustrating," Dale added, "that Paula's doctor pulled me aside and told me she would live only three to six months if we didn't do the full surgery, chemotherapy, and radiation treatments—the whole nine yards. My entire world stopped when I heard those words."

The doctor shook her head and sighed. "Doctors do *not* know how long you're going to live. It is insanely irresponsible to tell a patient how long they have to live. That is cruel and immoral. Many patients—thousands of patients—die each year because they believe the 'threat' their doctors give them. Doctors don't know. They can't know."

"If I knew then what I know now . . ." Dale stuck out his jaw, lowered his voice and growled, "I might have made him an offer he couldn't refuse."

"Don't worry, Doc. He's just kidding."

"I understand, Dale. He was wrong. But he learned, just as other doctors have, to give the patient a strong threat to motivate them to get them into treatment quickly. Otherwise, the patient may start searching for an alternative path. You see, the doctors are not running the show. Not like you might expect. Big business is in the driver's seat. And big business prefers that cancer patients get the expensive, drawn-out-care approach that brings in maximum dollars—not an approach of cancer prevention. Why? It's far more profitable for hospitals and healthcare professionals to have things drag on and on by creating a chronic condition than it is to cure the disease. As harsh as that sounds . . . cancer prevention? Ha! There's no money in that. No drugs? No doctor? No way!"

Kara's jaw dropped. This was a perspective she had not heard before. "Wow. That's shocking." She shook her head.

The doctor's words ignited a burning question in me. "Well then, how can I trust *anything* my doctor is telling me?"

"Believe me, I understand your concern, Paula. Most people have been programmed their entire lives to trust their doctor more than they do themselves. Most trust health professionals with their very lives. That's a problem. When people surrender their health care to someone else, no matter what credentials that person has, they are taking a huge risk. Especially nowadays. The general population doesn't understand that most doctors no longer think independently of the system. Protocols have been put in place for treatment of every disease and the doctors follow them like robots, almost without thinking. It's up to *you* to manage your own health care. Leaving it in the hands of someone else is dangerous, irresponsible, and often lethal. I'm not saying doctors don't have their place. They do. But only under *your* direction. You pay them, right?"

I laughed. "I'll say we do."

"Why do you have to do what they say just because they say it? Instead, pay attention to your body. Learn about health care for yourself. It's never been easier to do research than today. Basic college level study habits are more than enough. Aren't your health and life worth some focus and education?"

"Of course," I nodded. "So you're saying I need to treat doctors like mechanics. Ask for their diagnosis and recommendation and then do my homework and tell them what I want them to do."

The doc took a long sip of water before responding. "Yes, pretty much. Let me give you an example. Let's say your doctor says he'd like to remove your lymph nodes for inspection. Since the lymph nodes are an integral part of the immune system and your immune system will fight the cancer, you tell him no. It's as simple as that." She turned and wrote big letters on the board behind her: *NO.* "Paula, I am aware you have considerable swelling under your arm where the lymph nodes reside. Still I strongly recommend that you never allow anyone to remove your lymph nodes. They are swollen because they are trying to do their job . . . they are trying to stop the cancer from spreading.

"Next, let's say the doctor wants to do a needle biopsy on a lump in your other breast. Well, because tumors have many healthy cells in them, a needle biopsy does not provide enough tissue to determine accurately if the tumor is benign or malignant. You tell him no." She turned and underlined the word *NO.*

"Now, you may need to find another doctor, but, hey, he's working for *you*, right? You don't work for him. In fact, as his patient, you pay his bills. Bottom line—you need to manage your own health care. Especially right now but also for *all* the foreseeable future.

"You need to become an expert on how your body is designed to function. It's not difficult. It just takes some time and attention. Take time away from the many distractions of the world we live in. Time to read and learn and grow. Your life is worth it—am I right? Also, when you learn about your body, your immune system, and how your body fights disease, you'll understand why you need to avoid certain foods and toxins. And why you need to incorporate specific foods into your diet that contain the vitamins, minerals, and enzymes you need to live a vibrantly healthy life. Think how wonderful it will be never to worry about cancer. Think about having more energy than most people your age. Think about feeling good—and looking good—because you are living a lifestyle that keeps you disease free, just as God intended."

After a brief pause, Dale asked, "But what about the benign lumps in Paula's other breast? What should she do about those?"

"Look, any kind of a lump or cyst is abnormal. It is a warning sign. It can actually be a good thing *if* you heed the warning."

Kara's face scrunched up. "A good thing?"

"Yes, certainly. If you have a lump—*any* lump, benign or malignant—consider it a starter gun going off for a race. Now you race to change how you eat, drink, think, and live. Any lump is abnormal. It doesn't need to be cancerous for you to know that rebuilding your immune system is needed *immediately*."

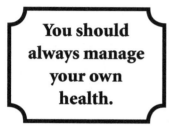

You should always manage your own health.

"What about the surgery Dr. Anderson is recommending on my cancerous breast? He couldn't get all of it. You know, the margins were not clear."

"If the cancer is already invasive and you have a large mass, it is sometimes acceptable to have surgery to get a jump start on getting rid of the mass. But what you need to remember is that whatever caused the cancer to begin with has to change or it will most likely come back—sooner or later."

"Having cancer return a second or third time is not an option I am willing to entertain. I'm scheduled for surgery in a little over a week—and then chemo and radiation right after that. I'm pretty sure I now know what you would recommend."

Dr. Cohen had periodically studied my medical documents throughout our discussion. Now she sat them down in an orderly pile and slid them back across the table toward me. "Don't ever let a doctor rush you into a decision. It's a game they play. Don't play it with them. Now about the surgery— I'm not completely against the mastectomy, but I don't think it is necessary. However, it is acceptable if you feel more comfortable taking that approach. At the same time, I do strongly recommend that you refuse the chemo and radiation now and forever. You have a large tumor already, which means you're very, very sick. You have signs that cancer has already spread. But don't panic when you hear me say that. It doesn't change anything at all for you.

"With cancer, you probably won't *feel* sick until it spreads to your organs and they start shutting down or the tumor gets so large that you have pain from the pressure it's creating. Believe me, Paula, you *are* very sick right now. Your immune system is *not* working or you wouldn't have a tumor.

"By now you know that pumping chemo into your already compromised body will destroy your immune system—and do long-term damage. Even though chemo kills some cancer cells because they're fast growing, it also kills healthy cells, including the fast growing cells of your immune system. If you don't strengthen your compromised immune system, you'll have no defense. And the serious staph infection that has required you to take antibiotics for weeks tells me your immune system is *completely* compromised. You need to start rebuilding your immune system immediately so your body can reverse the cancer."

"Doc, can chemo or radiation ever be used with a positive result for a patient?" Dale asked.

"Absolutely not. Chemo and radiation *cause* cancer. They devastate the immune system. No. Never."

"Okay, Doc. Then what should Paula do next? What's her best alternative course of action?" I could see Dale's anticipation growing. He wanted a solution as badly as I did.

"Yes, that's what I need to know now that I'm convinced I'm as sick as you say. What is the fastest way to build back my immune system and reverse the cancer?"

She smiled, sensing she had gotten the message across. "Okay, you two . . . I'm going to give you a quick overview today. You have a battle on your hands and you need to treat it seriously—and quickly. Don't delay. Every single day matters. And, Kara, you can be a huge help to your mother by supporting her and helping her with all she will have to do over the next several months."

Kara nodded. "I'm planning on moving back in with Dad and Mom to support them however I can."

"Good. That will help, especially in preparing the live foods and juicing ten times a day."

"Why does Mom have to juice ten times. Can't she juice less often and drink larger glasses?"

"Good question, Kara, but no. When someone is sick, they need a constant infusion of nutrients. It's the same reason a person takes antibiotics every so many hours instead of all at one time. Does that makes sense?"

Kara nodded. "I get it."

Dr. Cohen shifted in her chair. "Okay, let's talk about you getting well. First, God created you. He designed your body to function a certain way. God's plan is good and it works—we just have to get in harmony with it. There are two major components to getting well: what needs to go into the body and what needs to come out of it. Your immune system is healthy when you feed it the vitamins, minerals, enzymes, and water it needs to heal itself. These components also help your body detoxify. If you are sick or diseased, toxins build up in your body and constantly leak poisons into your bloodstream and cells. This keeps your immune system working overtime, attempting to rid your body of dangerous toxicity."

She looked right at me. "Paula, remember you brought this on yourself by not understanding what was causing the cancer now growing in your body. Now that you have learned *why* you have cancer, you—and only you—must take responsibility for what you now know. You are the only one who can reverse your cancer. None of us can do it for you. You will reverse it one day at a time. That's how you got it, and that's how you'll get rid of it.

"You must start by giving your body what it needs to have a strong immune system to fight the cancer."

"Would taking vitamins and supplements help?" I asked.

"That's not what I'm talking about, Paula. I *will* recommend some supplements, but I'm talking about *natural* enzymes and nutrients that you can get only from live food."

Kara sat up straighter. "What's *live* food?"

"Think of it as 'alive'—not dead food. Live food has not been tampered with but is in its natural condition, the way God created it. These foods have enzymes and nutrients that are 'super foods' for our bodies. They nourish our cells in ways that nothing else can—but only in their natural state. Cooking, freezing, or processing these live foods kills the enzymes, and you lose many, if not most, of the nutrients. You need living food for living bodies. Most of what people eat these days is dead food, which means it's cooked, canned, frozen, or processed. This leaves almost no nutritional value in the food, so your body receives worthless, empty calories. These types of dead foods may keep you alive for years, but they set you up for disease over time because your body is being depleted of what it needs to heal itself. You need living food for living bodies."

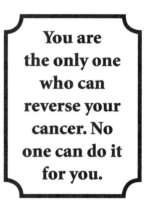

You are the only one who can reverse your cancer. No one can do it for you.

I reacted. "Wow. That describes much of the food we eat. I do have a salad now and then, and fruit once in a while, but most of the food I eat is cooked, canned, or frozen."

"Paula, that describes most of the western world. I'm going to guess that you use a microwave too. Is that right?"

"Yes. I use it a lot." I cringed. "You're going to tell me that's bad, aren't you?"

"Absolutely. First, it changes the structure of the food. It also puts radiation into the food you consume. So not only are you cooking, which kills nutrients and enzymes, but you're adding radiation to what you are eating, which further corrupts the food's value. It also puts radiation into the surrounding area. Of course, it's in small doses, but it all adds up."

"Oh, my goodness. Then what can I eat?"

"Because you are in a life-threatening crisis and have to turn your body around so quickly, you will have to be extreme in what you eat and drink for the next many months. It took you years to get this sick. It's going to take many months for you to get completely well again."

I was pretty sure I knew the answer to the question I was about to ask, but just in case . . . "What do you think about coffee or soda?"

"Absolutely not!" I cowered at the disgusted look that flashed across the doc's face. "You need to eliminate *all* caffeine, sugar, and artificial sweeteners as well as any canned or bottled drinks. They have no nutritional value and usually have chemicals and additives that are harmful. Caffeine is a diuretic. It actually depletes your body of water. Your body requires more water than is in the drink to neutralize the caffeine's effects. So caffeinated drinks literally cause dehydration, which is a huge contributor to getting cancer. Your body needs a lot of clean water to function normally and to grow new healthy cells. Drink only purified water with no fluoride or chlorine, natural fresh squeezed juice, or a limited amount of herbal tea without caffeine. Nothing more."

"But I'm already having headaches because I'm cutting back on the coffee and sodas."

I could see no sympathy as she shook her head and wagged her finger. "You need to get off those *now,* Paula. You do understand that this is your life we're talking about, right? You're in serious trouble. Let me say it again, based on what I've seen in your medical records and what you've told me, I'm going to guess that your cancer has already spread. You have to be extreme if you want to get well." She looked around the table at each of us. "Get extreme, kiddos.

"It's counterproductive to expect God to heal you if you continue to cause your problem. How can you pray and ask God to heal you when you then work against Him by violating the way He designed your body to function? It's no different from asking God to heal you of lung cancer while you're still smoking. But if you take responsibility to do all you can to help your body heal God's way, then I believe God will do whatever you cannot do and you will get well. That's how to reverse your cancer. One of the benefits of your Body-Soul-Spirit approach is that it will prevent sickness and disease from taking root in the future. A healthy immune system can prevent cancer as well as other diseases like diabetes, any autoimmune disease, heart disease . . . well, the list is endless. Here's the point: If you're healthy, you're healthy. Period."

"I know you're right, Doc," I agreed. "I need to get extreme."

"I'm glad to hear that. Now, do you have a juicer?"

"We have a blender. Won't that do the same thing?"

"No, that won't do. If you don't have a juicer, then buy one. Buy any juicer you can afford. I've seen people reverse cancer with all types of juicers. You need to be drinking at least ten glasses of fresh juice every day. Not store bought—fresh. That's your food for now. No meat, no dairy, and nothing processed or frozen. You should eat a bowl of oatmeal each morning, but use a milk substitute like rice milk or almond milk, however, not soy. Remember, no dairy—that also means no cheese or butter. I'm recommending eight carrot-apple juices and two green vegetable juices every day. I'll give you

> **It's counterproductive to expect God to heal you when you're the one causing the problem.**

some recommendations about what to include." (Details for juicing in Appendix B.)

Kara asked, "Can't she just eat the vegetables in salads and snack on carrots and apples?"

"No, absolutely not. When people have cancer, they need a tremendous amount of nutrients to rebuild their damaged immune system. There is no way you could eat enough vegetables to get all you need. Plus your body has to work hard to digest everything you eat, which taxes your body. Juicing is easy on your system and allows the nutrients to absorb quickly into your bloodstream. It's also the only way you can get all the nutrients you need into your body. You'll be juicing the equivalent of about twenty pounds of fresh organic fruits and vegetables every day. And by juicing so frequently, you will be continually feeding your body what it has been needing for years. This begins the healing process at the cellular level. Right where the battle is."

"Does that mean I don't eat anything else? What about protein?"

"You'll get plenty of protein from the vegetables you juice. It's incorrect to think you need meat or dairy to get protein. Everything you need is in natural vegetables— they're full of protein."

The information I was learning about the body was finalizing my Body-Soul-Spirit plan. I was getting some handles I could understand and control. My excitement was growing.

"While you are so sick, your primary food is juice. The only other food you should eat is oatmeal. You can snack on raw fruits and vegetables, preferably organic. If you can't find organic, than just wash them thoroughly to eliminate as many contaminants and pesticides as you can. But organic is far better for you. It has many more of the much-needed nutrients and enzymes than nonorganic foods."

"What about the four food groups or the food pyramid?"

Kara asked. "I remember learning about that in school. Doesn't Mom need other things to be healthy?"

Dr. Cohen shook her head. "Absolutely not, Kara. That is government propaganda to keep consumers buying from the various food industries. It's not what's best for you, believe me. If you want your mother to get well, she has to avoid those foods and replace them with whole, live, natural foods."

"Okay, Doc," Dale said. "We copy."

"Well, then, it sounds as though we're at a good place for a short break. How about we give ourselves fifteen minutes or so?"

Without missing a beat, Kara piped up, "Coffee anyone?"

We all laughed.

CHAPTER 18

Hard Questions Answered

*D*uring our break, Dale called to check on Jada but her daughter said she was too sick to come to the phone. Dale explained that we were meeting with a medical doctor who was helping me find an alternative path to reversing cancer and offered to ask the doctor about Jada's situation. The daughter freely shared details of Jada's condition and history, with Dale taking careful notes. Dale promised we'd get back to her after our meeting.

"Dr. Cohen," Dale said when our meeting reconvened, "Paula and I met a precious sister in the Lord who developed breast cancer three years ago. Her name is Jada and we love her dearly. She's fifty-two and has been having mammograms every year since age forty. They found a tumor, did a needle biopsy, and then performed a lumpectomy and removed several lymph nodes from under her left arm. Several chemo and radiation treatments followed. She and her daughter were grateful the cancer had been discovered early and were optimistic.

"Months later, near the end of her chemo treatments, she developed a blood clot near the chemo-infusion port on the inside of her arm, so she was given a drug called Coumadin for thirteen weeks. During the following years, she took Tamoxifen and Arimidex. Her daughter complained that these were of little to no apparent help.

"A couple of months ago, a mammogram revealed cancer in Jada's other breast. Her doctor, who by the way is Paula's doctor too, performed a mastectomy of her right breast and again removed several lymph nodes, this time from under her right arm. Since then Jada has been treated with both chemo and radiation again.

"She has also been suffering from a sluggish colon. Her doctor explained this condition is a normal result of the cancer, but it has plagued her for about three years. After her first bout with cancer, she had six colonic treatments and since discovering cancer again, she has had two more.

"Unfortunately, a CT scan (CAT scan—computerized tomography) now shows several tumors in her lung. She's having trouble breathing and experiences pain when she inhales. The CT scan also reveals small tumors in her lower back. In the last few days, she's experienced considerable pain when walking and now uses a wheelchair much of the time. She's gotten bad really fast."

Dale paused to scan his notes. "She has also taken two pain medications at different times—Dilaudid and Aredia. Jada is a strong Christian and still believes that God will heal her. She's been prayed for at church and, of course, we are praying for her too. She's a sweet, kind person with a tender heart and we've grown to love her . . . so this news is especially hard to take." Dale slid a piece of paper across the table toward the doc. "Here's a list of all the medications she's now taking."

"It's all happening so fast," I added. "She didn't seem that sick when we saw her a little over a week ago. Please, doc, can you tell us how to help our friend?"

Dr. Cohen's mouth tightened. "I'd like to begin by saying there *is* hope for Jada. It is quite late for her—but not too late to turn things around. Our God is a big God, and it is still possible for her to do what's necessary to become well. It's important that you three understand what has happened to your friend's immune system. It obviously would have been a lot easier if she had known the information I just finished sharing with you *before* she did these conventional treatments. Nevertheless, here's what I see has happened and is happening still."

Dale prepared to jot down notes as the doctor spoke.

"First, she's been having mammograms every year for nine years before she was diagnosed with the first tumor. You should know that each mammogram increases the risk of getting breast cancer. It's radiation. And in every mammogram, they usually take at least two x-rays. Anyone who has been having a mammogram once a year for roughly ten years has increased her chance of getting breast cancer exponentially."

I was shocked. "They say it's safe. I've always heard it's not enough radiation to be a problem."

The doc shook her head. "What else are they going to say? But it's radiation. Radiation is *never* safe—especially when you're exposed to it repeatedly. I am against having my patients get mammograms. Ultrasound is a better way, as it doesn't use radiation. But the best way, as far as I'm concerned, is a manual inspection by a physician.

"So let's continue. Three-plus years ago, they discovered a tumor and Jada had a lumpectomy. As you know by now, for her to have a tumor reveals that her immune system was already seriously compromised—which is why she developed cancer in the first place. After her lumpectomy, she underwent radiation and chemotherapy treatments, doing further damage to her immune system and increasing her chance of getting more cancer. All the while, these treatments dramatically decreased her body's ability to fight the cancer. Several of her lymph nodes were removed. As you now know, lymph nodes should never be removed. They are an integral part of the body's immune system and are critical in helping to prevent cancer from spreading.

"You say she developed a blood clot in her arm from her chemo port. This is no surprise and fairly common. Many of the drugs she has been taking contribute to an increase in blood clots. In addition, dehydration is a major cause of cancer and some of the drugs she's been taking have the side effect of—wouldn't you know—dehydration. Most cancer patients don't eat enough high-water-content foods or drink enough water. Dehydration causes the blood to thicken and therefore tend to form clots. You mentioned she was given the blood thinner Coumadin. This drug, like all synthetic drugs, has many side effects, some of which can even be fatal. I won't go into detail, but I would be remiss if I didn't say that one possible side effect is hemorrhaging into the brain. Other less serious side effects include the destruction of skin or other tissues, edema, fever, rash, dermatitis, fatigue, vomiting, diarrhea, and hair loss."

My head was swimming with all the new data. I felt as if I were at the receiving end of a conveyor belt of information that wouldn't slow down. I shook my head, trying to refocus.

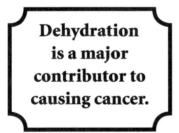

Dehydration is a major contributor to causing cancer.

The doctor glanced at the paper Dale had passed to her and continued. "Her daughter mentions she is taking the drugs Tamoxifen and Arimidex. Tamoxifen is literally poisonous and so, of course, represses the immune system further. It can also cause uterine or liver cancer. As we know, the liver is an important organ because it is the detoxifying organ. Tamoxifen does serious damage to the liver's ability to rid the body of toxins and disease. Then there's Arimidex, which also has several destructive and serious side effects like excessive blood clotting, low white blood cell count, joint pain, muscle pain, anxiety, nervousness . . . should I go on? All these things contribute to exactly what the patient does *not* need and does *not* want. Good grief. The other drugs you mentioned are no different. Remember, drugs don't cure disease. Drugs only treat symptoms. And synthetic drugs have many side effects. Their risks outweigh any benefits.

"Then, more recently, Jada had her right breast and more lymph nodes under her right arm removed. She underwent more chemotherapy and more radiation. Unfortunately, as we've discussed, although chemotherapy and radiation destroy some cancer cells, they also destroy good cells. And many of these good cells are cells of the immune system. And didn't I mention . . . the immune system is the *only* system that can fight cancer."

We nodded. I was hearing things I had read or heard before, but each time the information sank in a little deeper. I was having to replace a lot of old learning. "Please continue, Dr. Cohen. Not only will we share this information with Jada, but it's helping me to hear it too."

Dale's hand was scribbling notes at lightning speed as he tried to keep up.

Dr. Cohen took a long sip from her water bottle before continuing. "The daughter also mentioned that Jada's colon is sluggish and so she has had multiple colonic treatments. This is not surprising. The culprits here are likely the pain medications she's been taking and dehydration. One of the primary reasons cancer develops in any person is that the body cannot eliminate waste materials fast enough. This is usually because of side effects of the meds or a lack of water, fiber, and exercise. The colon slows down and the toxins the body needs to expel remain in the body and begin to be reabsorbed into the bloodstream. This is a serious condition that must be corrected immediately. Usually, however, it goes unchecked. The colonics will not likely improve the sluggishness of her colon. Instead, she needs to drink a lot of water and, as I've been explaining to you, she should be drinking large amounts of fresh vegetable juice and eating a diet high in fiber. It is imperative that she eliminate all dairy and all meat immediately from her diet. I have to say, it is very late for Jada—but it's not *too* late."

Jada had become an integral part of my life. We were dealing with cancer and life and death together. My voice trembled. "Wow, Doc, her condition sounds so serious. Do you *really* think she can still turn things around?"

"Yes, Paula, I do. But she has to stop doing all the things that are making her circumstances worse. The daughter said the CT scans now show several tumors in her lungs, as well as several small tumors in her lower back. This is highly unfortunate but predictable with her treatment background. Her cancer has metastasized. If you think about it, why wouldn't it have spread? Every treatment she's had has been counterproductive to her healing. None of her treatments deal with the root of her cancer. A few *temporary* indicators along the way may have showed her cancer was not growing, but with the conventional treatments she has undergone, these indicators are generally short-lived. Radiation and chemotherapy cause cancer—they cannot possibly reverse it. These treatments have severely reduced her natural ability to resist cancer, which is why she is in such dire condition now.

"Her doctors and her family have the wrong perspective about cancer. They seem to be convinced that cancer, like some foreign invader, has attached itself to her body and is spreading." With a deep sigh, she continued. "This way of thinking is completely backward. There is no long-term hope if a person continues to treat the tumor as if it's the cancer.

"I don't mean to sound harsh, but the truth is that Jada gave herself cancer gradually, over time, by the way she eats, drinks, thinks, and by the way she lives. She has done exactly what you and I both did, Paula. People cannot get rid of cancer by further destroying their immune system. What Jada must do now is reverse the factors that caused the cancer in her body in the first place. She needs colossal amounts of nutrition consistently poured into her body immediately. She needs to hydrate her body continually. She needs to eliminate stress, anxiety, and worry. Of course, that will be more difficult now, considering her present condition. She needs peace, love, joy, hope, and faith. She needs to think about and talk about healing and health and vibrant life. She needs to sing and laugh and bathe herself in the love of God. All while she is juicing ten times each day and eating a vegan diet as well as doing all the other things I've shared with you. You cannot get rid of cancer by further destroying your immune system.

"Let me add this in closing. Please brace yourselves. Jada has no possibility of recovering from her condition with conventional medicine. Standard treatments may delay the outcome, but without changing things at the root level, eventually she will be another victim of the medical system."

I felt as though I'd been kicked in the stomach.

The doc continued. "Jada's doctors—your doctors, Paula—will give her more and more of the same. They'll give her more chemo, more radiation, more surgeries, and more drugs. They'll drain as much money from her insurance as possible. They'll continue these destructive treatments until they suck so much life out of her body . . . well, until there's no life left. The only chance Jada has to reverse the enormous damage that's already been done to her is to quickly rebuild her immune system by natural means. Nothing else can possibly save her."

The room was silent. My heart knew that what the doc had shared was true. Still, it was a tough prognosis. *Will there be time for Jada? Will she be willing to do what is needed in the eleventh hour?*

The quiet was broken when a uniformed pilot stuck his head in the room. "Doctor, your aircraft is ready."

"I'll be right there." She turned back to us. "Paula, Dale, Kara, it has been a pleasure meeting with you." Fixing her eyes on mine, she added, "Paula, I believe you know enough now to get well. Remember . . . follow your plan. You're right. It *is* spirit, soul, and body—all three parts working together in harmony with God. Your approach will bring you through. You need to combine spiritual principles with the natural laws of health. And by the way, you cannot give your approach just a serious attempt. Intense military discipline—that's what you'll need. Put more effort and more energy into your approach than anything you've ever done in your life—it will take that kind of devotion. And it *is* that important.

"Others with stage IV cancer have reversed it with alternative means. You may at times feel as if you're on a roller coaster, but stay the course. Keep praying. Keep believing God has brought you your way of escape. Fight the good fight of faith. If you do—I believe you'll be victorious."

My eyes welled up with tears. Never in my life had I been more challenged.

"Would you like to pray together?" the doc asked as she stood.

The four of us moved into a close circle and held hands as Dr. Cohen led us in a heartfelt prayer for divine understanding and for the touch of God's healing power on my body.

I have to be able to see her again—or at least talk to her.

"What's the best way to communicate with you, Doc? How can I reach you again?"

"Listen, kiddos, you don't need me now. You have found your way. You won't need to reach out to me again. Keep your gaze on God. Stick to your Body-Soul-Spirit approach." She placed a gentle hand on my shoulder. "Stay the course, Paula. You found your way of escape. Now, all of you, follow your plan." She turned and walked toward the door.

And then she was gone.

CHAPTER 19

Life Choices

⟫

*T*he clock read 9:30 a.m. Though stunned that I'd slept so long, I smiled at how rested I felt. My new lifestyle required it; alarm clocks were banned. Previously my M.O. had been to stay up late and get up early. I'd taken pride in how much I accomplished each day—how many hours I worked. Unknowingly, I had lived most of my adult life in a sleep-deprived state.

Since learning that the all-important immune system uses sleep time to repair itself, I'd slept as long as I wanted, without guilt. Leisurely stretching under the covers, I enjoyed the lack of pressure. *So nice. I could get used to this.*

Jada! The memory of Jada's worsening condition flooded in. *I need to tell her about what God has shown me.* Jolting out of bed, I quickly dressed and headed toward the phone. I arranged with Jada's daughter for Dale and me to visit that afternoon.

Dale and I pulled up to Jada's house, and I watched for her to come bounding out the front door. This time, no one appeared.

No smiling face, no warm hug of greeting. My heart sank. Jada's daughter escorted us into a dimly lit living room. Shades were drawn—the interior devoid of sunshine. The air was stagnant. An old movie played on a muted TV. Scattered across the top of the coffee table were plastic prescription bottles—no doubt pain medications. Jada was lying on her side on the sofa under a thick wool blanket. She struggled to sit up.

Moving to her side, I placed my hand on her arm. "Oh, Jada, don't try to sit up. Just relax. It's so good to see you, sweetheart," I whispered.

"Hi, Paula. Hi, Dale. It's good to see you too." Her voice was shaky and weak.

Dale and I were both taken aback by her visibly frail condition. Her eyes, which had always been bright and full of life, were flat, with none of their usual luster.

I gave her a long warm hug. Her body was smaller than the last time I'd wrapped my arms around her. "We're so sorry to hear the news, Jada." I was having trouble accepting how quickly she had declined. *How could all this have happened in only ten days?*

Jada insisted, so I helped her sit up, propping pillows behind her back. Tears trickled down her cheeks. "I know I've gotten a lot worse, but I'm still gonna beat this thing." Tenderly grasping my hands, "I've really missed you, Paula—missed our talks." We leaned toward each other until our foreheads met. For several moments, we sat locked in place.

Jada filled us in on her new symptoms. "They're using *much* stronger chemotherapy this time around. It makes me sicker than ever. Plus, I'm getting radiation on my back to try to shrink those tumors. Wow, I'm so tired. I have no energy at all. It's especially difficult the days just after my treatments."

I cringed. She was following medical protocol to the letter. Her doctors were my doctors—we used the same hospital. Up to this point, our paths had paralleled. Not anymore.

Though eager to share my new discoveries, they now seemed out of place. I squirmed in my chair.

Then Jada asked, "Where have you been, Paula? How are you doing?"

I paused and then decided it was time to tell her what I had learned. I told her about God's promises and my way of escape. I talked about our research, the books, the videos, our new understandings about cancer, and the miracle meeting with the doctor. Then I shared a detailed description of the Body-Soul-Spirit approach to reversing cancer. I was passionate . . . excited. I couldn't help talking as if I'd found buried treasure.

During my discourse, Jada's eyes glazed over. I had hoped for a positive response. It never came.

Jada forced a weak smile. "I'm happy for you, Paula, but I can't change course now. I trust Dr. Anderson and Dr. Marcus, and they believe there's hope for me. And I still believe God will heal me through these treatments. Lots of people are praying—I'm not giving up."

"Mom's doctor said we should start to see some results very soon," Jada's daughter interjected. "We can't stop the treatments now. The doctor wouldn't allow that. They promise that the chemo and radiation are Mom's best chance of knocking out her cancer."

I tried to hide my disappointment. Jada was deeply entrenched in the medical system and so sick she could barely think clearly. Between the doctors, the drugs, and her daughter, Jada was losing control. She was in serious trouble. The situation was heartbreaking.

Before heading home, we held hands and Dale led us in prayer. We drove much of the way home in silence. Tears trickled down my face now and then—and I could feel the knot of dread in my stomach. *Lord, Jada needs a miracle now—to change the way she's thinking. Please help her. Please.*

For the next two weeks, I was immersed in my new

lifestyle—literally betting my life on my Body-Soul-Spirit approach. I trusted God daily. In order to *trust* Him, one must *know* Him. Thankfully, I did know God—personally and intimately. He was my Salvation, my Healer, and my Provider.

Each day I made sure I held no anger, resentment, or lack of forgiveness in my heart. I learned that for me to get well, I could not allow those destructive emotions. Nor could I allow myself to wallow in self-pity. I began to think of myself as an overcomer—already healed—already cancer free. Controlling my thoughts consistently proved to be one of my biggest challenges, but it was a hurdle I eventually overcame by quoting Bible promises, praising God for my victorious outcome, and speaking faith-filled affirmations. We called these things "heart-talk."

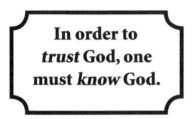

In order to *trust* God, one must *know* God.

Anger, resentment, and lack of forgiveness are destructive emotions that prevent healing.

The "Body" part of my approach was easiest. It was logical and out in the open. Much of it was what I *wouldn't* eat or drink, as well as what I *would* eat and drink to nourish my body and repair my immune system. The cornerstone of my new diet was juice—fresh organic vegetable juice ten times every day—eight glasses of carrot-apple juice and two glasses of green vegetable juice. (See Appendix B for several of my juice recipes.) Juicing also kept me from getting hungry. If I snacked, it was on raw vegetables or a little fruit—nothing more. And each morning I ate a bowl of oatmeal.

I focused on taking in the vital nutrients my body needed for healing, while denying myself anything that would compromise that process. Every day I also drank twelve eight-ounce glasses of pure, clean water—free of fluoride, chlorine, and other harmful contaminants.

To stop the damage to my immune system, I eliminated

common offenders like sugar, caffeine, coffee, and soda. Meat and dairy products were banned entirely. Nothing cooked, fried, or frozen was allowed. No fast foods or processed foods passed my lips. It took a while to get through the withdrawals and cravings, but the outcome was worth the cost. I was becoming more comfortable with my new lifestyle every day.

Dr. Anderson had scheduled my surgery and was expecting me in his office in a couple of days. My decisions could be put off no longer.

Admittedly, I was shaken by Jada's condition. I had tried to suppress the realization that deadly cancer was growing in my own body, but seeing Jada had renewed my awareness of the severity of the unrelenting threat.

Something else happened that shook me to my core. I called the four other women in my cancer club to find out how they were doing and to share my discoveries. Donna's cancer had spread to her brain. Sherry's cancer had spread to her lungs. They were both back on the cancer treadmill—more chemo, more radiation, and more drugs. Unfortunately, my new approach garnered no interest. Cancer is about life and death. Cancer is also about choices.

> **Anger, resentment, and lack of forgiveness are destructive emotions that prevent healing.**

I needed help sorting things out concerning my looming surgery and treatment options. After sharing the latest news with Dale, I asked, "Can we talk about what I'm going to do?"

"Absolutely, sweetheart. Of course. What would you like to discuss?"

"Dale, I'm so out of time. Every day . . . every hour . . . counts. I've always known cancer is lethal, but it has become more of a threat now as I see it devastating the lives of my friends. Here's my thinking. I will *not* have the chemo treatments. I'm also against radiation. It's quite obvious to me now that adding dangerous poison or devastating radiation into my body is contradictory to God's original design. It's contrary to His way of healing."

"Oh, Paula, I'm so relieved. Whew. I completely and wholeheartedly agree." Dale's body relaxed. Then he asked, "How are you feeling about surgery in light of all that is happening to your friends?"

"The surgery is where I'm stuck. I remember Dr. Cohen saying that in my case surgery was acceptable, even though she didn't believe it was necessary. But gosh, Dale, after seeing how bad Jada has gotten so fast . . . after hearing about Sherry *and* Donna . . . I must say, it's paralyzing. On top of that, let's not forget that Dr. Anderson could not remove the entire cancerous tumor last time. That knowledge weighs heavily on me." I paused and took a deep breath. "I'm also struggling with guilt. Even though I was aware of the lump in my breast, I let it go unchecked for over a year. Of course, I regret it now. Foolishly, I allowed cancer to grow in my body for a long time."

> Cancer is about life and death. Cancer is also about choices.

"I know it, honey. Darn it. But we have to share the guilt. We just figured it was another benign cyst like you'd had in the past. We now know that *any* tumors—even benign ones—are warning signs."

"True. But there's more, Dale. The other symptoms I'm dealing with indicate my cancer has spread—the lump on my arm is growing, the lymph nodes are swollen and increasing in size, and the pain in my abdomen is getting much worse. Well, putting it all together, it's downright overwhelming. I'm committed to staying the course. I've got to follow my escape plan plus do anything and everything I have the ability to do.

Bottom line is, I know I need to trust that God will make my way of escape crystal clear."

"Paula, let me say that in all you do, let's not forget that it's your *life* that is most important. You must live to fulfill the plan God has for you. And dying before your appointed time doesn't line up with Bible promises, nor does it line up with how we are praying. We need to make decisions based on whatever gives you the best chance of living . . . with or without body parts. And may I add something else?"

"Of course."

"Well, I wasn't going to bring this up unless I felt it could be beneficial . . . but now, maybe it can be."

"What are you talking about?"

"Paula, when we were in San Diego, the doctor pulled me aside and told me she was quite convinced that your cancer has spread. She felt it would help me to know this so I could add my influence to keep you following your lifestyle changes to the letter. Because you're following your plan with extreme discipline, I wasn't going to bring it up. But now you're at a big crossroads. Maybe knowing what the doc said can help you."

"Wow." I paused and gazed out the window, taking in this new piece of information. "Thank you for telling me, but that's not a huge surprise. Okay, Dale, let me ask you point-blank. How would you feel if, for safety's sake, I had both my breasts removed? You should know that's what I'm considering." I held my breath and waited.

"Honey, your life is what I care about . . . not your breasts. I want *you* . . . with or without breasts. I love *you* . . . not your body. I mean, it's your choice . . . and I'll support whatever you decide to do. I just want you to live. I also want to see you stay in line with God's Word and His ways."

"Thank you, Dale. That's how I thought you'd feel, but it's also what I needed to hear."

As difficult as the previously aborted surgery had been,

I could now see God's divine intervention in delaying that surgery long enough for Dale and me to learn all I needed to know in order to make the decisions I needed to make. I felt like a different person in the same body.

The next morning Dale and I were ushered into an exam room where Dr. Anderson greeted us with a smile. "Paula, are you ready for surgery tomorrow?"

Swallowing hard, I responded, "Doctor, I've made the decision to only allow limited surgery—a double mastectomy, but I don't want any of my lymph nodes removed. They are an essential part of my immune system so I need them. And I'm rejecting all radiation and chemotherapy treatments. We've done a tremendous amount of research, and I believe God is leading me this way. I've carefully thought this through and it's *exactly* what I want to do." I braced for his retort.

He paused and crossed his arms. "Paula, I must tell you, I do *not* agree with your decision." He opened my file and scanned the pages in silence. Then, looking directly into my eyes without a blink, continued. "You and Dale have done a lot of homework and I know that you aren't making this decision flippantly. So, even though this is against my professional recommendations, I will respect your wishes."

I exhaled and my body, rigid with tension, relaxed. "Thank you."

"Well then, I'll see you at the hospital in the morning. Remember, no food or drink after midnight." He turned and briskly walked out of the room.

Dale and I looked at each other. "Whew. He was not happy about my plan."

"No, he wasn't, Paula. But he agreed." Both of us were certain Dr. Anderson knew if he hadn't complied with my request, I would have walked out and found a doctor who would do what I asked. I was now firmly in charge of my own health care.

When I walked out of the hospital a few days later, I made a promise to Dale—and myself. "Dale, I am now done with the medical system in my battle with cancer. I will not be back. There is nothing more they can offer me that I want. Even if I get sicker and look like I'm getting real close to losing this battle, I'm *not* coming back. Through thick or thin, I'm committed to following the plan God has given me—my Body-Soul-Spirit approach."

I had drawn a line in the sand. Each day I focused unwaveringly on my new lifestyle. My self-discipline had never been stronger, but my symptoms continued to get worse, not better. The lump on my arm grew larger. The pain in my abdomen got more severe. Some days, I couldn't walk at all. My faith was challenged by my circumstances and crippling fear at every turn. Despite my challenges, I didn't waver. I didn't buckle under the pressure. I stayed the course.

TWO MONTHS LATER

Kara and I walked into the house from my trek around the block. The walk had been painful and drained all my energy, but with Kara's help, I had succeeded. Dale met us at the door. One look at his face and I knew something had happened.

"What's wrong, Dale?"

He stepped back and gazed out the window, then quietly uttered, "Oh, my word. Houston, we have a problem."

"Oh, no. What is it?"

Dale sat down, his body tightly contained. "Paula, honey. Kara. Brace yourselves."

"Why? What's happened?"

"I answered a call from Jada's daughter a few minutes ago."

"No. Oh, no."

"Sweetheart, Jada died this morning."

For several heartbeats, there was not a sound in the room. The news had shocked me into silence. I sank into a chair. *How could Jada be gone?* "Oh, dear Lord, no!"

Dale lowered his head and for several moments stopped breathing. I stared at the floor, my thoughts somersaulting over every conversation Jada and I shared over the last couple of weeks. I could feel her arms around me the last time we hugged. I could still see her thousand-watt smile from better days. I could feel her hair brushing my cheek when we last said good-bye. Now those arms . . . that hair . . . that smile . . . were gone. Though I knew there was always a chance that neither she nor I would beat cancer, I could not come to grips with the reality that Jada had lost her battle.

Jada was gone. Gone from this world. Gone forever.

Chapter 20

End of the Road

Three months had passed since Jada's memorial service. Every day I threw myself into my new lifestyle with military discipline. I had forgone the chemo and radiation treatments entirely and refused all drugs for pain. I hadn't deviated from my plan even once in those three months, but . . . I'd gotten worse. The pain in my abdomen increased so much that taking walks was no longer possible. The lump on my right arm continued to grow. The swelling under my left arm increased. Day after day, my faith was put to the test by circumstances and symptoms of deterioration. Every twinge of pain invited fear—relentless fear that hounded me like a hunting dog following a scent.

By this time, however, I had a well-established battle plan firmly in place. When fear showed up, I would pull out my handwritten Bible promises and read each verse aloud with strong conviction. I affirmed those promises with an alert mind and an open heart. Not one time did I skip even a single scripture. Although I knew the verses well, I needed to speak them—needed to hear them—over and over.

I faced this struggle to overcome fear with faith several times each day. Whenever doubt or anxiety came charging in, I would pull out my three dog-eared pages of promises and go on the offensive. In the same way light pushes out darkness, hope and faith expelled the fear. It was the most difficult battle I had ever faced—the battle of a lifetime. Through it all, my self-discipline never wavered—there was too much at stake. My very life depended on it.

Dale was fighting a battle of a different kind. Instead of turning to those in our church for help, Dale got a job and worked as much overtime as he could to provide the things I needed. He pulled away from people and drew intimately close to God, a behavior he had honed after the airplane crash to gather strength for his spirit.

With only one source of income, we struggled to pay our normal expenses plus the medical bills that came in from my three surgeries and doctors' visits—the bills my insurance would not cover. Soon we were buried in financial challenges and medical debt. Sometimes it felt as though our lives had been turned upside down and dumped out of a box.

It took about eight months of rigorously following my lifestyle regimen for my body to respond. But eventually . . . I could tell that my immune system was getting stronger. Little by little. Step by step. My energy began to increase. Finally the lump on my arm began to melt away. The swelling under my arm slowly disappeared. It took longer for the pain in my abdomen to subside, but after a few more months, it too gave up its hold and gradually diminished until it was gone.

It took about fifteen months to really feel good again. I looked good too—healthy and vibrant. At least that's what everyone around me said. There was a glow about me. My hair had a sheen I'd not seen since my youth. My body was slim and trim and I could again walk without pain. I felt like I did in my twenties.

I was not the same person I had been when my journey started—not spiritually, not emotionally, and not physically. Although I was showing encouraging signs every day, I was reminded of how lethal my battle with cancer was when I heard the news that both Donna and Sherry died of the disease—only weeks apart. Eventually, all five women in my cancer club—the five women whom I had befriended and had come to respect and love—all succumbed to cancer. I alone survived.

TWENTY MONTHS AFTER MY CANCER DIAGNOSIS

I hadn't seen Dr. Anderson since my last surgery. His office had sent me countless letters over the last eighteen months urging me to return. I had ignored them all. But now I *wanted* to go back. Was my cancer gone? With one phone call, Dr. Anderson had willingly agreed to arrange a full-body scan. With great apprehension, I returned to the familiar medical facility for the test.

Two days later Dale and I were escorted into Dr. Anderson's personal office to receive the test results. We took seats facing his desk. I studied his face for clues as he entered the room and sat down.

"Hello, Paula. Hi, Dale. It's nice to see you both again." Dr. Anderson flashed us a tentative smile as he fidgeted with his pen. "We've tried several times to reach you. I'm glad you decided to come back and see me. How are you feeling, Paula? You're certainly looking good."

"Thanks, Doc. It's nice to see you too. I'm feeling great actually. In fact, I feel healthier and stronger than I have in years."

I could see my medical file lying on his desk. *The test results must be in there. How long is he going to keep us waiting?*

After a few more pleasantries, Dr. Anderson opened the folder but continued to look directly at me. "I have good news, Paula." He paused before continuing. "I'm happy to report that you are completely clear of cancer." He smiled broadly. "There is no sign of any abnormality. Congratulations, both of you. Paula, you are cancer free."

Sitting stone still for several seconds, I let the words *cancer free* sink in. Unaware of the degree of pressure that had been building inside me, tears began cascading down my cheeks as the tension broke. I helped myself to several tissues from a box on the desk before throwing my arms around Dale's neck. For several moments, no one uttered a word.

Emotions were thick. Dale reached to grab his own fistful of tissues. Slowly shaking his bowed head, he wiped his eyes and nose. Dr. Anderson shifted uncomfortably in his chair. Then Dale looked up and smiled, breaking the tension. "How much do we owe you for the box of Kleenex, Doc?"

Dr. Anderson laughed.

Dale wiped his eyes repeatedly, finally mumbling, "Well, thank the good Lord!"

Dr. Anderson shook his head. "Dale, Paula, I'm not sure what to actually make of all this. I'm not sure what you did, Paula. I know you refused chemotherapy and radiation treatments. You may have found another doctor. But whatever you did, you obviously did the right thing."

Though I still couldn't find words to speak, my mind was doing cartwheels. *God is faithful! He is so faithful! He showed me my way of escape. How would I have ever done this without You, Lord? Thank You. Thank You. Thank You!*

Dr. Anderson's words interrupted my thoughts. "Paula, if you don't mind, I'd like to hear what you did. I'd like to know how you got well. You may remember my mother. Her cancer has returned with a vengeance and now has spread to her brain."

Dale and I sat with Dr. Anderson and shared my Body-Soul-Spirit approach. We recounted all I had done to get well. Although reluctant to show signs that he agreed with our methods, he listened intently for the better part of an hour.

Back in our car heading for home, we were both overcome with jubilation. Dale honked the horn and shouted inside the car. Then he rolled down his window and screamed into the desert wind like a teenage girl at a rock concert. Still, that wasn't enough. He detoured onto a sandy desert road, got out of the car, and yelled and hollered some more. I grinned as I watched.

My joy was over the top. As the news sank deeper, I became more and more excited. I leaned over and honked the horn, accompanying Dale's screams. My heart felt like exploding out of my chest. Boundless, intoxicating joy welled up inside me.

I watched as Dale punched the air with his fists. I got out and jumped and sprinted and kicked the sand and laughed out loud. I laughed and laughed and laughed.

Then Dale and I put our arms around each other and leaned against the car, watching the late afternoon sun slide below San Jacinto Peak. My heart overflowed with joy. *Pinch me*, I ordered my guardian angel. I still could hardly believe this was real.

> **God will use anything for your good and His glory—*if* you do things His way.**

It's truly official now. I have to believe it. I do not have cancer.

Cancer had been my life's greatest challenge. Although cancer had never defined me, the journey certainly did. I learned that God would use anything for my good and His glory—*if* I did things His way. God's Word proved itself again and again. The Bible *is* the only truth I can find in this crazy, mixed-up world.

My heart leaped when I remembered the day God gave me a personal promise. Just loud enough for Dale to hear, I whispered the sacred words, "God will not tempt you beyond that which you are able to endure . . . without making a way of escape."

Overcome with emotion, Dale could only nod in agreement.

God was true to His promise.

I had found my way of escape.

The End

APPENDIX A:
Body-Soul-Spirit Approach
by Dale

Overview

When most people think of sickness or disease, they think only about the body. But according to the Bible, God created all people in His likeness—in three parts: *body*, *soul*, and *spirit*. Each of these parts plays a different role, yet they interconnect. Each has a great effect on health or sickness, life or death. This means that even when sickness or disease is apparent in your body, the illness may be rooted in your spirit or your soul. Thus, for permanent vibrant health, you must address all three parts—your spirit, your soul, and your body.

The *spirit* refers to your spiritual heart, not your physical heart. You *are* a spirit being, created in God's image. God is a spirit. The *real* you is your spirit, not your body or mind.

You also have a soul, consisting of your mind, your will, and your emotions. Though it's probably the least understood of the three parts, the soul has a profound effect on your life in a myriad of ways. People commonly believe the soul and spirit refer to the same thing—but they do not. According to Scripture, they are clearly different, yet both are eternal parts of your being.

You live in a body that exists to house your spirit and soul. Your body allows you to interact with the physical world in which you live. The body is the easiest part to understand because you can see it and touch it. You can literally feel your body, inside and out. For example, if your toe hurts or your head aches, you know your body is afflicted. Your body is also the part of you that others acknowledge and with whom they interact. If you don't consciously adjust your way of thinking, you can get stuck believing that your body is who you are. But your body is where you live—not who you are. You—the *real* you—is your spirit.

Think of your car as an example. It's the vehicle you use to get around. When people who know you see your car coming, they say, "Here comes so-and-so." They recognize you by the car you drive, but you are *not* your car. Similarly, you need a physical vehicle—your body—to carry your spirit and soul through this natural world. In summary, you *are* a spirit, you *have* a soul, and you *live in* a body.

Because each of these three parts interconnect and interrelate, one part cannot be affected without the other parts responding either positively or negatively.

Let's discuss each of the three parts as it relates to sickness and disease. Then I will share with you what Paula did to reverse her cancer.

Spirit

The most important part of the Body-Soul-Spirit approach for Paula was knowing for sure that if she died of cancer she would go to heaven to live with God. At last check, the death rate is still 100 percent—we will all die sometime. But since so many die every year of cancer (more than half a million in the U.S. alone), Paula needed to revisit her beliefs about life after death and determine whether she was *prepared* to die. (For more information about life after death, visit "Book Your Heaven Flight" at http://daleblack.org/book-a-heaven-flight.asp .)

It is your spirit, which the Bible also refers to as your heart, that interacts with God. You process that interaction with your mind and can express it with your body. Your spirit is developed by giving attention to the things that feed it—things like reading God's Word and spending time with Him in prayer. Prayer is simply talking with God. Problems can originate in your heart and then affect your health in a big way. Attitudes like unforgiveness, resentment, and envy are rooted in the spirit but have a profound impact on your physical health.

Another important part our spirit plays in dealing with sickness is recognizing that the Bible is God's Word. *His Word is the source of life.* Spending time in prayer and reading the Bible were paramount in helping Paula find the path that was right for her and determine what was true. *God's Word is truth.*

Confidently believing that God wants you well is the cornerstone of the faith needed to trust Him for healing. The specific promises Paula used to strengthen her faith and dispel fear can be found in Appendix C.

Certainly God can heal supernaturally. Paula and I have experienced the miraculous personally plus we've watched miracles occur in lives of others around us. But, for a myriad of reasons, God more often uses a *combination* of spiritual truths *and* natural laws to bring your entire being into alignment with His will. Paula realizes that if God had answered her prayers for healing with an instantaneous miracle, it would have been only a matter of time before she was sick with cancer or some other chronic disease again. God wanted her (and me) to learn His ways and to walk in complete truth and health by bringing our spirit, soul, and body into agreement with His design.

Often people get angry with God if He doesn't provide them a miracle healing. And most of these people do not even look for another option. But God is a big God, a good God. He wants us to mature and learn more about Him and His ways.

I know Paula well, and I watched her every move when she had cancer. I knew what she was thinking much of the time. Without question, Paula knew God wanted her well. Once she found her "way of escape," she didn't look back. Paula often says, "When I die it will *not* be from disease. Jesus revealed God's will when He healed *every* sickness and *every* disease in His day. He works the same today as He did then." How could she be so strong and determined? Because she believed the Bible. She spoke Bible promises aloud with conviction several times each day. She trusted in God's Word and walked in agreement with it.

What God did for Paula, He can do for you. God's Word *is* more certain than your circumstances. Paula prayed for a miracle healing from her advanced cancer, but it didn't happen that way. We began looking for what else God wanted her to learn. Just as He showed Paula her way of escape, He will show you your way of escape too—if you'll trust Him and seek His direction diligently. Remember that a relationship with God is a partnership. It takes two—Him and you.

Paula prayed and asked God to heal her. She had the elders of our church anoint her with oil and pray for healing according to the scriptural promises found in James 5:14 and Mark 6:13. Then she found others with faith who agreed to pray for her. Everything she could do according to Scripture, she did. Then she continued praying and reading the Bible, looking for God's direction.

God could have supernaturally healed Paula at any time—she was always expectant. But she didn't just sit and wait—she took action. She continued to seek truth and understanding. It didn't take long before Paula learned she could change the way she ate, drank, thought, and lived. She constantly searched for what more she could do—what adjustments God may want her to make. Let me assure you, if you or a loved one has been diagnosed with cancer or another chronic disease, change—major change—is required.

Soul

Your soul is also an eternal part of your being. Some refer to it as your personality. The soul is made up of your mind, your will, and your emotions. You have the power to renew your mind—and the Bible instructs you to do just that. "And do not be conformed to this world, but be transformed by the renewing of your mind, that you may prove what is that good and acceptable and perfect will of God" (Romans 12:2).

Everything about your soul begins with the way you think. This renewing process starts with new thinking based on the truths in God's Word. Once you learn a new truth, you must put it into action in your life. This is accomplished by using your will. Your emotions will follow just as the caboose follows the engine on a train.

The mind is a powerful part of the soul and needs to be guarded and treated intelligently. Understanding the difference between *truth* and *knowledge,* and learning to sift *truth* from *information* is a lot like panning for gold.

Effective cancer-fighting strategies use the mind, the will, and the emotions. Your mind will be renewed as you discover new truths. You will be "changing your mind" when these new truths replace what you previously believed. Your emotions will follow your new actions.

How you think of yourself is vital. If you are sick, do you think of yourself as a victim? Do you struggle with self-pity? These common dangers have serious consequences.

Allowing others to show you special treatment can be intoxicating—but it can also be deadly. Once you believe you are healed, then you must act in a way that agrees with what's in your heart.

Turning away extra attention was a difficult decision for Paula to make, but she knew that she must refuse to be identified as a cancer patient. She never saw herself as a member of the "cancer club." And afterward, when she was pronounced "cancer-free," she would not allow herself to be called a "cancer survivor." She refused to connect her identity in any way to being sick or diseased.

No matter how sick you may feel, or how sick your doctor has said you are, it is imperative that you visualize a long and bright future. Make plans that are motivating and talk about them with expectancy. Talk regularly about reaching your future goals. Paula did not build "pipe dreams," but she did develop *real* faith for a *real* future for her life and health—rooted solidly in God's Word.

Another part of the soul is your *will*. Learn to use your will to make right choices. Decide now that when you find truth, you will not waver—you will take a stand.

Emotions are an important, yet potentially dangerous, part of the soul. If you have not learned to evaluate and harness your emotions, you can easily be derailed with feelings rather than truth. Feelings and emotions *do* matter, but they should never control you.

Negative emotions like anger, panic, and fear create physiological stress on the body. These damaging emotions release stress hormones into the bloodstream that further weaken your immune system. If negative emotions continue unchecked, they can destroy a person's immune system, even if that person is doing everything else right. Regularly evaluate yourself. Are you harboring negative emotions? Permanent health and healing are not possible if negative emotions are continuously present.

Body

As previously mentioned, the body is the easiest of the three parts to understand because it is the most visible. You use your body for seeing, hearing, and touching, as well as moving and interacting with others. Sickness and disease manifest in the body; therefore, we must also deal with the illness at the body level. But the body is only a part of the whole you. To become well and stay healthy, you must address all three components—spirit and soul and body.

When sickness shows up, many go to their doctor for help first. But in fighting chronic disease, including cancer, Paula and I sadly discovered that the medical system is broken and upside down. Neither chemotherapy nor radiation treatments cure cancer. Drugs don't cure disease.

Doctors treat symptoms, not root causes. In Paula's battle with cancer, we learned that doctors are taught to cut, poison, or burn out tumors with surgery, chemotherapy, and radiation. But none of these methods treat the cause of cancer—they only deal with the tumors. Yet tumors are *not* the cancer. Tumors are the *symptoms* of cancer. The patient may sometimes show temporary signs of improvement from chemotherapy and radiation; however, those treatments deplete and destroy the immune system, making the cancer worse at the root level—not better. In Paula's case, her doctors didn't deal with the reasons her cancer developed in the first place, something Paula discovered she would have to do herself.

NEW LIFESTYLE

When Paula was diagnosed with cancer, there was no time to lose in making big changes. We realized that God created our bodies to heal themselves and if we would honor His design, the body would heal naturally and stay healthy.

Below are many of the principles Paula (and I) followed. They explain how she got her life back.

Avoiding Stress

Avoiding stress was essential. Stress has many harmful effects on the body and damages the all-important immune system. Paula's main challenge was recognizing and avoiding the many sources of stress. It comes in many forms and is often labeled an "invisible killer." Stress can show itself either physically or emotionally, and both can cause physiological damage.

Some of the more common root causes of stress are lack of sleep, pressure at work or from people, relationship issues, financial pressures, toxins from food or drink, toxins from the environment, drugs, dehydration, insufficient oxygen, and lack of nutrients coming into the body.

Stress creates an oxygen deficiency in the blood and a release of stress hormones into the bloodstream. Oxygen deficiency causes shallow breathing and constricted muscles and blood vessels. Lack of oxygen in the cells is known to be an underlying cause of cancer. Stress hormones can increase the growth rate of cancer and feed existing tumors, causing them to spread.

The human body fights off disease primarily with white blood cells. During times of stress, the body releases corticosteroid, a hormone that can lower the number of lymphocytes (a type of white blood cell) in the body. This lessens the body's ability to fight off foreign agents such as cancer cells.

For Paula to have less stress, she had to quit working. Giving up that source of income caused other stresses, but we made choices together about which things were most important. Paula believes that leaving her job was one of the decisions she had to make in order to relieve her stress and adopt her new lifestyle. Material things don't mean much when measured against life and death.

Rest

Adequate rest is paramount. The immune system repairs and recharges during the rest cycle. Our bodies are designed with a distinct natural cycle called the Circadian rhythm. This natural cycle includes light versus dark—day versus night. Keeping the body on this natural cycle is an important part of producing good hormones and less stress.

As Paula eliminated stimulants like sugar and caffeine, her sleep improved. She no longer set an alarm clock but slept until she wanted to wake up. For years she had deprived her body of the rest she needed, so it was time for payback. She was finally getting enough rest, and at the proper time of day.

Oxygen

As I previously mentioned, oxygen is a critical component to healthy cells. If cells are oxygen deficient, they become vulnerable to cancer and other disease. Paula increased her oxygen levels with exercise—she took walks daily for as long as her health allowed. We learned that certain foods contain higher amounts of oxygen, and they became part of her daily regimen (see Appendix B for juicing recipes). Cancer starts at the cellular level; therefore, having healthy, oxygen-rich cells (red blood cells carry oxygen to our tissues) increases our immune system's ability to destroy cancer-causing damaged cells.

For the first time in her life, Paula started to breathe properly. She took long slow deep breaths. She did this in the cleanest air available. We tried to leave a window open at home when possible. Paula learned that she needed a proper balance between negative and positive ions in the air that she breathed. Too many positive ions typically exist in places like office buildings, gymnasiums, and church buildings, and the air is therefore unnatural. This is caused when heating and air-conditioning units remove many of the negatively charged ions in the air, causing fatigue, dizziness, and headaches. Studies have shown that an increase in negatively charged ions inhibits the growth of cancer tumors. So Paula's new lifestyle involved breathing good *quality* fresh air throughout the day.

pH Balance

Lab studies suggest that cancer cells thrive in an acidic (low pH) environment but cannot survive in alkaline (high pH) surroundings. A person's pH is a measure of how acidic or alkaline that person is. A pH of zero is completely acidic and a pH of fourteen is completely alkaline. A pH of seven is considered neutral and desirable. A person's pH can be determined with a simple litmus strip in the mouth. These strips can be purchased online or at any local drugstore. As Paula continued her new lifestyle, juicing, and eating naturally healthy foods, the pH in her body balanced itself automatically. Instead of focusing on her pH, Paula focused on her new lifestyle. Her pH, therefore, was never a concern.

Water

One of the first things Paula and I implemented in our new lifestyle was drinking twelve 8-ounce glasses of water every day. Just any water wouldn't do—it had to be clean bottled or filtered water (not tap) without chlorine and without fluoride.

Water regulates all human body functions. We use water for breathing, perspiring, and digestion. Our cells need hydration to function properly and to keep our immune system working at an optimum level. Inadequate hydration is a frequent cause of cancer and many other diseases. Moreover, when someone doesn't get enough water, pain is often the result. Proper hydration can even help a person suffering from arthritis, including rheumatoid arthritis.

Since our body is made up of 75 percent water and our brain 85 percent water, Paula began hydrating herself to the point we thought she might float away. She even got additional water by juicing the high water content vegetables every day.

Sunlight

Sunlight causes an increase in negative ions, which slows the growth of cancer cells and promotes vitamin D. Both are needed to fight cancer and other disease.

For years we had heard that we should stay out of the sun to avoid skin cancer. Certainly, we should not bake in the sun to the point of sunburn, but for thousands of years human beings on this planet have been exposed to the sun with little damage. Once we learned the benefits, Paula tried to get about thirty minutes of natural sunlight every day. Being outdoors also helped with another need—clean oxygen.

Nutrition: Juicing

In modern Western society, the standard diet is grossly deficient for providing the amount of nutrients our body needs to heal itself. Paula got cancer because, in simple terms, her immune system was not working properly. To provide her with massive amounts of the right nutrients quickly and consistently to bring her back to health, we turned to juicing. The human body is designed to heal itself if nourished properly. Paula needed to do her part to help her body perform the way it had been designed by God to function.

The fastest and best way to nourish the cells in Paula's body was for her to drink fresh organic juice ten times every day. Her juicing schedule and the recipes she used are found in Appendix B.

Fresh juice should be consumed only on an empty stomach, allowing the vitamins and minerals in the juice to go straight into the bloodstream. Ideally, Paula drank her juice immediately after preparation. As soon as the juice is exposed to air, its live enzymes begin to degrade, destroying some of its nutritional value.

Blending is *not* the same as juicing. When you blend, pulp and solids remain in the juice. These solids inhibit the juice from being absorbed directly into the bloodstream and instead send it through the digestive system.

Paula's primary juice was carrot and apple. Carrots are high in carotenoid content, which is shown to help prevent and reduce cancer. They are also rich in vitamins A, B complex, C, E, and potassium. The apples sweetened the carrots as well as adding additional nutritional benefits. Apples are rich in phytonutrients and bioflavonoids. They contain vitamin C, which is an antioxidant that helps protect the body from infectious disease and helps reduce toxicity. Apples are also rich in beta-carotene, which boosts the immune system. Paula drank eight 8-ounce glasses of carrot-apple juice every day.

Check with your local health food store as many of them carry large twenty-five pound bags of organic carrots at a reasonable price. If you cannot afford organic, buy regular. Though nonorganic are not as rich in nutrients and may have some chemical contaminants, people have reversed cancer with nonorganic carrots as well.

Paula preferred to prepare and drink fresh juice every hour. But another option is to juice once for the entire day and store the juice safely so it doesn't lose too much of its nutritional value. The juice must be kept cool in a tightly contained thermos or sealed jar. Some value will be lost by storing, but there are times when it's helpful to juice once for the day, such as when you need to be away from home.

Besides the carrot-apple juice, Paula drank two 8-ounce green vegetable juices each day. Many high nutrient value vegetables feed the body and cells. Many vegetable drinks can also include apples for sweetening. Apples are the only fruit that can successfully be mixed with vegetables in juicing.

Supplements

Paula took daily supplements of organic green barley, which she occasionally substituted for the green juice. Daily, she also took a natural multivitamin, large doses of Ester C several times throughout the day, additional antioxidants, and flaxseed oil.

Avoid Meat and Animal Products

Paula stopped eating meat—beef, chicken, fish—all of it. We learned that the human intestine is not designed for these foods. It takes the human body about three days to digest meat. Because it stays so long in the intestines at body temperature, it putrefies, releasing toxins into the bloodstream. Meat often contains harmful pesticides and hormones, which add toxins to the body. Paula committed to eliminating all meat from her diet until she was completely well.

Many people mistakenly believe they need meat for adequate protein; however, there is more than enough protein in vegetables to provide all a person needs.

Avoid Dairy

Paula gladly eliminated milk as well as all dairy from her diet—no cheese or butter. Dairy is animal protein and fat, which needlessly tax the immune system.

Avoid Cooked and Processed Foods

When food is tampered with and taken out of its natural form, it is no longer "living" food. Heating food eliminates the beneficial living enzymes and most of the nutrients. Baked, fried, or barbecued foods are the biggest offenders. These methods of cooking form toxic compounds and kill off most of the food's nutrients. In addition, vitamins are water-soluble, and a significant percentage is lost in cooking. Many plant enzymes that function as phytochemical nutrients in our body and maximize health can be destroyed by overcooking.

Gently steamed vegetables and homemade soups are acceptable in moderation as a supplement to raw foods and juicing. Though some nutrients are lost with conservative cooking, others are made more absorbable. When gently heated, many vegetables and beans provide additional nutritious compounds that would not be absorbed by eating them raw.

When vegetables are steamed or made into a soup, the temperature should be fixed at 100 degrees Celsius or 212 Fahrenheit—the temperature of boiling water. This moisture-based cooking prevents food from browning and forming toxic compounds. Acrylamide, the most recognized of the heat-created toxins, is formed only with dry cooking and not with boiling or steaming. Many essential nutrients in vegetables are made more absorbable after being cooked in a soup, and water-soluble nutrients are not lost because we eat the liquid portion of the soup as well.

Processed foods are foods that have been altered from their natural state for convenience and storage. These foods are packaged, canned, boxed, or bagged and have been cooked, dehydrated, or preserved in some way. They contain chemicals and additives such as sugar and high fructose corn syrup, MSG and other flavor enhancers, aspartame, sodium, potassium benzoate, sodium nitrate and nitrites, artificial food colors, along with a host of other substances that are harmful and to be avoided.

Juicing was the foundation of Paula's diet and provided most of her intake. She also added some raw foods (salads, raw fruit, and vegetable snacks) lightly supplemented with gently steamed vegetables or homemade soups.

Avoid Microwaving

Many people use microwaves to cook or heat food. This was a convenience Paula gave up immediately. Microwaving changes the structure of the food, plus it releases radiation into the food or beverage as well as the surrounding area. Radiation causes cancer. Even though a microwave emits a low dose, it all adds up over time. Paula eliminated every toxin she could control.

Avoid Caffeine

Eliminating caffeine was a difficult adjustment for Paula because of her addiction to it, but she eliminated all caffeine in all forms from her diet immediately. Learning how adverse the effects of caffeine were shocked her to reality. Caffeine constricts the arteries, increases blood pressure, worsens diabetes, promotes food allergies, creates fluid retention, and contributes to cancer of the bladder, cancer of the ovary, and breast cancer. Caffeine also robs the bones of calcium and causes dehydration.

Studies indicate that daily use of caffeine reduces calcium of the bones by 14 percent each decade. In other words, twenty years of drinking one or two cups of coffee a day increases calcium loss by 28 percent. This is shocking but true. We were stunned to learn that ten grams of caffeine is considered a lethal dose—approximately seventy cups of coffee in a day. People have actually died by ingesting too much caffeine in a 24-hour period. Caffeine and alcohol are diuretics; they leach water out of the body.

Avoid Refined Sugar

When Paula learned how devastating and damaging processed sugar is, she understood why it needed to be eliminated from her diet. Almost every processed food found in today's market contains sugar. Sugar robs the body of calcium, zinc, chromium, vitamin C, and vitamin B complex. It liberally coats the cells of the immune system for approximately four hours, which prevents the immune system from reacting to the presence of any cancer cells. That meant Paula would lose four hours of cancer fighting after ingesting sugar. Not only that, but sugar or high fructose corn syrup actually *feeds* the cancer cells.

Sugar triggers the body to release the feel-good hormone serotonin, but once the effects wear off, it causes irritability and confusion, depression, and excessive tiredness. Sugar is considered by many to be toxic to the body and causes a myriad of problems. It wears on the pancreas, leads to diabetes, and produces insulin in the body. Sugar also promotes tooth decay and hair thinning and weakens the bones. It robs the body of oxygen, which is essential for healthy cells. There is nothing beneficial about ingesting refined sugar.

Sugar substitutes, most often found in diet drinks and sugar-free foods, are even worse. The most dangerous by far is aspartame, which also goes by the names of NutraSweet and Equal, among others. According to the FDA, 75 percent of adverse reactions from food additives are associated with aspartame. The more serious conditions associated with this additive include brain tumors, Alzheimer's, Parkinson's, multiple sclerosis, migraines, and birth defects.

Avoid Drugs and Chemicals

Prescription and over-the-counter drugs add chemicals and toxins into the body, further stressing the immune system. Chemicals in foods, like additives and artificial sweeteners, are toxins that drain the immune system. Previously, Paula took pain killers regularly for headaches and even prescription medicine for migraines. But once she properly hydrated, eliminated caffeine and aspartame, and greatly reduced her intake of salt, the headaches that had plagued her virtually disappeared.

Fluoride is a dangerous chemical found in toothpaste and mouthwash. Americans have been convinced that fluoride will save their teeth, and we drink fluoridated water more than any other nation on earth. Studies have been done showing fluoride as a poison that accumulates in our bones. It has been associated with cancer in young males. It causes osteoporosis, reduced I.Q., and hip fractures in the elderly—just a few of the many problems it causes.

Aluminum, a dangerous metal, is in deodorant. These two harmful substances—fluoride and aluminum—are in products most people use every day. Paula threw away her toothpaste and deodorant and started using natural products only. She eliminated the dangerous chemicals and metals lurking in so many cosmetic and hygiene products. We learned to read the labels on everything.

Paula's Daily Schedule

Below you will find Paula's typical daily schedule of what she ate and drank to help reverse her cancer. Once Paula determined her course, just after we met with the doc, she never looked back. I never heard her complain about what she couldn't eat and never saw her cheat—not even once. She was diligent in following her new lifestyle. Her life depended on it and she knew it. She also knew that God had revealed His natural way of healing, and she wanted to be faithful to what God had shown her.

If Paula wanted a hot beverage, she drank hot water with lemon as often as she wanted—and occasionally herbal tea. This counted toward her minimum of 96 ounces of water every day.

For breakfast she ate a bowl of hot oatmeal (no microwave), adding raw honey to sweeten, and Rice Dream or almond milk in place of regular dairy milk. Beware of the instant oatmeal that often contains additional substances like fake fruit or sugary additives. The only oatmeal that is acceptable is the type cooked on the stove in boiling water—the old-fashioned way.

Paula and Kara (sometimes I helped too) prepared fresh juice every hour between 9:00 a.m. and 6:00 p.m. Eight of these servings were carrot-apple; the other two were green juice.

We became accustomed to drinking juice during the day, and lunch was always carrot-apple juice for everyone while Paula was rebuilding her immune system. Even after she was completely well, we continued to drink carrot-apple juice for lunch and for an afternoon snack.

Because Kara and I still wanted to eat solid food for dinner, Paula would often join us with a salad full of fresh organic vegetables (lemon juice for dressing) and occasionally some steamed broccoli or another vegetable. This never replaced her juicing, so she was seldom hungry for any other food.

We learned not to mix fruit and vegetables in the same meal (except when juicing with apples) because they digest at different rates. Fruit must be eaten on an empty stomach since fruit travels through the stomach more quickly than other foods. If fruit is eaten with any other foods that digest slower, it tends to ferment in one's system and release toxins, which can be harmful.

In Summary

God created and designed your body to be fueled by the foods He provides. These foods are natural and alive. God never intended His creation to live on artificially manufactured food with almost no nutritional value and filled with dangerous chemicals and additives. Is it any wonder that we are a sickly and obese nation? Only living foods packed with God-given nutrients can rebuild a person's disease-fighting immune system.

FREE GIFT - Paula's "Jump Start Plan"
Jump start your health with your FREE GIFT (valued at $30).
Receive one Healthy Juice Recipe, one Faith-Building Bible Promise,
and one "Heart-Talk" Affirmation from Paula
by email EVERY DAY for 30 days.

Send email to: jumpstart@lifecancerandgod.com

APPENDIX B:
Juicing Recipes and Other Tips
by Paula

There are many sources of juicing recipes and almost unlimited possible combinations. However, in this section I will discuss only some basic understanding of juicing and provide the recipes I used when I had cancer.

Organic vs. nonorganic. It's true that organic foods are more expensive than nonorganic; however, if you can afford it, the benefits of organic far outweigh the few dollars' difference.

It all starts with the soil. Nonorganic soil uses fertilizers containing three primary nutrients—nitrogen, phosphorus, and potassium. But healthy soil *should* contain over fifty nutrients. Poor soil health leads to poor plant health because the plants draw their nutrients from the soil. If the soil is deficient, the plants are deficient. Because of deficient soil, the plants are not as naturally pest and disease resistant, so they are sprayed with pesticides, herbicides, and fungicides to keep them healthy enough to sell at market. When we eat nonorganic food, we not only eat food deficient in nutrients, but we also ingest harmful chemicals that have compromised the plants as they have grown.

Studies show that organic soil has higher levels of zinc, boron, sodium, iron, and more. Organic soil also enhances a number of biological properties such as enzyme activities and micronutrient levels. Depending on the specifics of the farm or other location where the produce is grown, the organic benefits can range from moderately better to abundantly better in nutrient richness. Not only is organically grown food healthier, but it also consistently tastes better.

I recommend organic whenever possible, especially if you

are sick and juicing to get your health back. You will be ingesting a large amount of produce. If you juice nonorganic food, the potential increase of chemical bombardment to your immune system could be detrimental.

Whenever possible, buy local produce. Reducing transport time limits the possibility of contamination and bacterial growth. Also, nutrients in fruits and vegetables start to break down as soon as they are harvested. The three natural destroyers of vitamins and nutrients in produce are light, heat, and oxygen. Proper storage can prolong the life and nutrient level of your food.

Why and how to wash your vegetables. Fresh produce can harbor bacteria, fungi, and other microbes along with trace amounts of chemicals—wash it well. Always start with clean hands, clean countertops, and clean cutting surfaces.

Wait until you are ready to use it to wash your produce. Wash it under running water slightly cooler than the temperature of the produce. If you are soaking, use a bowl rather than the sink, as the sink often harbors bacteria. Do not use detergents or bleach to wash produce since it is porous and might absorb harmful contaminants.

For leafy green vegetables, separate and wash leaves individually, discarding outer leaves if they are torn or bruised. Leaves can be difficult to clean sufficiently, so immersing them in a bowl of cold water for a few minutes will help loosen contaminants. Follow with a cool-water rinse. After washing, prop in colander to drain or pat dry with paper towels. If you are using the leaves for juicing, additional moisture does not have to be removed.

Juicing vs. blending. Juicing and blending are not the same thing, nor do they provide the same result. The great value of juicing is that the nutrients are absorbed directly into the bloodstream within about twenty minutes, bypassing the digestive system. Juicing gives you maximum nutrient absorption with the least amount of stress on your body. In contrast, blending retains the pulp and solids, making it necessary for the substance to travel through the digestive system. This takes hours instead of minutes and requires your body to work harder with slower and less absorption of the needed nutrients.

When I had cancer, if I had eaten the amount of vegetables and fruit I juiced, I would have had to chew and digest approximately twenty pounds of food a day—and would still not have received the benefits I received from juicing. Eating instead of juicing is simply not practical when you are trying to get well.

The top nutrient-rich foods I used in my juices are listed below, along with their incredible benefits.

Carrots. This superfood provides antioxidants from carotenoids, including beta-carotene. Antioxidants have anticancer properties and protect the arteries. They act as an antiseptic and diuretic, boost immunity, work like an antibacterial, lower blood cholesterol level, and prevent constipation. Carrots are also rich in vitamins A, B-complex, and C; iron; calcium; and potassium. They help cleanse the liver and digestive system, help prevent kidney stones, and relieve arthritis and gout. Carrots also enhance mental function and decrease the risk of cataracts and macular degeneration.

Carrots are easily storable and remain fresh for up to two weeks if stored in a cool place such as the crisper drawer of your refrigerator. Cut off the green tops as soon as possible because they continue to draw nutrients from the carrots. Do not juice the tops. The carrots will stay fresher if you do not wash them until you are ready to juice. Note: Since I bought large twenty-five pound bags, I used an ice chest for storage and kept them cool with several blue ice containers, which I replaced twice a day.

Apples. Fresh apples help clean the system and eliminate toxins. They lower blood cholesterol, maintain blood sugar levels, and aid digestion. Apples contain vitamins A, B, C, and riboflavin and are high in pectin and boron—two important phytochemicals (compounds that may affect health).

For juicing, apples are versatile. They are the only fruit that can be mixed with vegetables without negative effects. (Fruits and vegetables contain different enzymes for digestion, and apples are the only neutral fruit.) They can be added to carrot and green juice equally well and contribute a sweetness or tartness, depending on the apple type. Do not juice the seeds.

Apples range from sweet to tart. Select your apple for the taste you want. Fuji, Sonya, Gala, Jonagold, Cameo, Golden Delicious, and Red Delicious apples are sweet (listed most sweet to least sweet). Granny Smith, Jonathon, Pink Lady, Braeburn, Rome, and Honey Crisp apples are tart (listed from most tart to least tart).

Kale, Swiss chard, collard greens, Romaine lettuce. These leafy greens are strong sources of vitamins A and C, chlorophyll, and some calcium, iron, folic acid, and potassium. They are excellent antioxidants and anticancer.

Spinach. Known for its anticancer properties, spinach also improves memory and promotes healing. It is anti-cataracts and anti-anemia.

Celery. This vegetable provides a wonderful base for several varieties of green juices. It is a mild diuretic and contains anticancer properties. Beneficial in combating high blood pressure, it also helps detoxify carcinogens.

Cucumber. The cucumber's high water content makes it another wonderful base vegetable for green juice recipes. It acts as a mild diuretic and contains vitamin A, iron, and potassium.

Paula's Juice Recipes

Carrot-Apple Juice
5–8 carrots (depending on size)
1 sweet apple

Lively Green Juice
4 stalks celery
3–4 leaves of kale
1 green apple

Green Popper Juice
1 cucumber
2–3 collard leaves
2 sprigs fresh parsley*
1 green apple

Green Beet Juice
Several leaves of Romaine lettuce
1 cup fresh spinach leaves
1/2 beet
1 sweet apple

Sweet Green Juice
2 carrots
2–3 collard leaves
3–4 kale leaves
1 sweet apple

See additional juicing options on next page.

Optional additions to any of the juices, depending on personal preference:

(The measurements given are per serving.)

Ginger (1/2 inch)
Garlic (one clove)
Green bell pepper (1/2)
Beet (1/2—1)
1/2 lemon
Parsley (2 sprigs)*

*Individuals with kidney or gallbladder problems may want to avoid eating parsley.

Try different combinations of these healthy ingredients. Find the ones you like best or make up your own version. All the ingredients listed are full of healthy nutrients and will help you regain your health and stay healthy. Enjoy!

FREE GIFT - Paula's "Jump Start Plan"
Jump start your health with your FREE GIFT (valued at $30).
Receive one Healthy Juice Recipe, one Faith-Building Bible Promise,
and one "Heart-Talk" Affirmation from Paula
by email EVERY DAY for 30 days.

Send email to: jumpstart@lifecancerandgod.com

APPENDIX C:
Healing and Faith Scriptures
by Paula

God's Word is health and life.

"My son, give attention to my words; Incline your ear to my sayings. Do not let them depart from your eyes; Keep them in the midst of your heart; For they are life to those who find them, And health to all their flesh. Keep your heart with all diligence, For out of it spring the issues of life." (Proverbs 4:20–23 NKJV)

God's Word will never expire.

"Heaven and earth will pass away, but My words will by no means pass away." (Matthew 24:35 NKJV)

"But the Word of the Lord (divine instruction, the gospel) endures forever. And this Word is the good news which was preached to you." (1 Peter 1:25 AMP)

We need God's Word to sustain life.

"Man shall not live *and* be upheld *and* sustained by bread alone, but by every word that comes forth from the mouth of God." (Matthew 4:4 AMP)

Success requires trust in God.

"Roll your works upon the Lord [commit and trust them wholly to Him; He will cause your thoughts to become agreeable to His will, and] so shall your plans be established *and* succeed." (Proverbs 16:3 AMP)

Your choice matters.

"I call heaven and earth to witness this day against you that I have set before you life and death, the blessings and the curses;

therefore choose life, that you and your descendants may live." (Deuteronomy 30:19 AMP)

God's benefits include healing.

"Bless the Lord, O my soul; and all that is within me, bless His holy name! Bless the Lord, O my soul, And forget not all His benefits; Who forgives all your iniquities, Who heals all your diseases, Who redeems your life from destruction, Who crowns you with lovingkindness and tender mercies, Who satisfies your mouth with good things, so that your youth is renewed like the eagle's." (Psalm 103:1–5 NKJV)

God's Word is healing.

"He sent His word and healed them, And delivered them from their destructions." (Psalm 107:20 NKJV)

God wants you to live.

"I shall not die, but live, and declare the works of the Lord." (Psalm 118:17 NKJV)

God promises His children a long life.

"With long life I will satisfy him, and show him My salvation." (Psalm 91:16 NKJV)

Jesus bore your sins AND your sickness.

"But He was wounded for our transgressions, He was bruised for our guilt *and* iniquities; the chastisement [needful to obtain] peace and well-being for us was upon Him, and with the stripes [that wounded] Him we are healed and made whole." (Isaiah 53:5 AMP)

You must take authority over the sickness in your body.

"Assuredly, I say to you, whatever you bind on earth will be bound in heaven, and whatever you loose on earth will be loosed in heaven." (Matthew 18:18 NKJV)

Agree with someone for your healing.

"Again I say to you that if two of you agree on earth concerning anything that they ask, it will be done for them by My Father in heaven." (Matthew 18:19 NKJV)

Have the elders of your church pray for your healing. (Make sure they believe in healing and follow the instructions in the Bible.)

"Is anyone among you sick? He should call in the church elders (the spiritual guides), and they should pray over him, anointing him with oil in the Lord's name." (James 5:14 AMP)

What you *believe* matters.

"Therefore I say to you, whatever things you ask when you pray, **believe** that you receive them, and you will have them." (Mark 11:24 NKJV, emphasis mine)

What you *say* matters.

"So Jesus answered and said to them, 'Have faith in God. For assuredly, I say to you, whoever **says** to this mountain, "Be removed and be cast into the sea," and does not doubt in his heart, but **believes** that those things he **says** will be done, he will have whatever he **says**.'" (Mark 11:22–23 NKJV, emphasis mine)

Fear is not from God . . . rebuke it!

"For God has not given us a spirit of fear, but of power and of love and of a sound mind." (2 Timothy 1:7 NKJV)

Cast down thoughts and imaginations that don't line up with the Word of God.

"For the weapons of our warfare are not carnal but mighty in God for pulling down strongholds, casting down arguments and every high thing that exalts itself against the knowledge of God, bringing every thought into captivity to the obedience of Christ." (2 Corinthians 10:4–5 NKJV)

We can have confidence He hears our prayers and answers.

"And this is the confidence (the assurance, the privilege of boldness), which we have in Him; [we are sure] that if we ask anything (make any request) according to His will (in agreement with His own plan), He listens to *and* hears us. And if (since) we [positively] know that He listens to us in whatever we ask, we also know [with settled and absolute knowledge] that we have [granted us as our present possessions] the requests made of Him." (1 John 5:14–15 AMP)

"And whatever you ask for in prayer, having faith *and* [really] believing, you will receive." (Matthew 21:22 AMP)

Obey God.

"We ought to obey God rather than men." (Acts 5:29 NKJV)

What is faith?

"Now Faith is the assurance (the confirmation, the title deed) of things [we] hope for, being the proof of things [we] do not see and the conviction of their reality [faith perceiving as real fact what is not revealed to the senses]." (Hebrews 11:1 AMP)

We live by faith.

"For we walk by faith, not by sight." (2 Corinthians 5:7 NKJV)

Establish your faith for your healing.

"So faith comes by hearing [what is told], and what is heard comes by the preaching [of the message that came from the lips] of Christ (the Messiah Himself)." (Romans 10:17 AMP)

"He personally bore our sins in His [own] body on the tree [as on an altar and offered Himself on it], that we might die (cease to exist) to sin and live to righteousness. **By His wounds you have been healed.**" (1 Peter 2:24 AMP, emphasis mine)

"And a great multitude came to Him, bringing with them the

lame, the maimed, the blind, the dumb, and many others, and they put them down at His feet; and **He cured them**." (Matthew 15:30 AMP, emphasis mine)

"And Jesus went about all the cities and villages, teaching in their synagogues and proclaiming the good news (the Gospel) of the kingdom and **curing all kinds of disease** and every weakness and infirmity." (Matthew 9:35 AMP, emphasis mine)

"And all the multitude were seeking to touch Him, for healing power was all the while going forth from Him and **curing them all** [saving them from severe illnesses or calamities]." (Luke 6:19 AMP, emphasis mine)

"Bless the Lord, O my soul, And forget not all His benefits; Who forgives all your iniquities, Who **heals all your diseases**." (Psalm 103:2–3 NKJV, emphasis mine)

"Jesus Christ is the same yesterday, today, and forever." (Hebrews 13:8 NKJV)

"Fully satisfied and assured that God was able and mighty to keep His word and to do what He had promised." (Romans 4:21 AMP)

"I call heaven and earth to witness this day against you that I have set before you life and death, the blessings and the curses; therefore **choose life,** that you and your descendants may live." (Deuteronomy 30:19 AMP, emphasis mine)

FREE GIFT - Paula's "Jump Start Plan"
Jump start your health with your FREE GIFT (valued at $30).
Receive one Healthy Juice Recipe, one Faith-Building Bible Promise,
and one "Heart-Talk" Affirmation from Paula
by email EVERY DAY for 30 days.

Send email to: jumpstart@lifecancerandgod.com

APPENDIX D:
Affirmations
by Paula

My confessions of faith—or affirmations—were a powerful part of keeping my faith strong, stable, and focused. Faith cannot be silent or still. It always requires agreement, action, and risk. If you have nothing to lose, you don't need faith.

If I need something from God, my responsibility is to pray and diligently search God's Word for direction. If I truly believe God wants me well, I need to take action to walk according to the truth He has revealed. Then I reinforce my belief continuously in my heart, in my ears, and with my mouth. I do this with affirmations based on scripture. The three scriptures below are guidelines for using affirmations.

> "Assuredly, I say to you, whatever you bind on earth will be bound in heaven, and whatever you loose on earth will be loosed in heaven." (Matthew 18:18)

> So Jesus answered and said to them, "Have faith in God. For assuredly, I say to you, whoever **says** to this mountain, 'Be removed and be cast into the sea,' and does not doubt in his heart, but **believes** that those things he **says** will be done, he will have whatever he **says**." (Mark 11:22–23, emphasis mine)

> But **be doers of the Word** [obey the message], and **not merely listeners** to it, betraying yourselves [into deception by reasoning contrary to the Truth]. For if anyone only listens to the Word without obeying it *and* being a doer of it, he is like a man who looks carefully at his [own] natural face in a mirror; For he

thoughtfully observes himself, and then goes off and promptly forgets what he was like. (James 1:22–24 AMP, emphasis mine)

Affirmations are like proclamations. I speak what I believe in my heart and give God's Word authority in my life through what I proclaim. I choose to line myself up with life and health, not death and sickness. What I don't say is just as important as what I say.

During my battle with cancer, once I was convinced I knew God's will for my situation, I committed my course to action. From that time on, I never spoke again that I was sick, or had cancer, or that I might die. I only spoke what I was believing for. That doesn't mean negative, fearful thoughts never entered my mind—in fact, they plagued my mind regularly. But I made a choice. I knew I could not walk or speak in faith *and* doubt at the same time and still get the result I was believing for. My scriptures and affirmations kept my faith strong and my goals focused on getting well and living a long life.

When I am fighting negative circumstances like cancer, I know it may take time for the physical realm to change course and agree with what I am believing and establishing in the spiritual realm. In my battle with cancer, I was committed for however long it took to experience the physical confirmation of my healing. I had faith that if I did everything God had revealed to me, He would do whatever I could not. I love Ephesians 6:13 in the Amplified translation: "Therefore put on God's complete armor, that you may be able to resist and stand your ground on the evil day [of danger], and, having done all [the crisis demands], to stand [firmly in your place]." I was going to stand firm and do all I could do—for as long as it took.

It's important to understand that affirmations, or proclamations of faith, don't change God—He never changes. It is always His will for you to be healed. But affirmations do change you. Continuously speaking words of faith helps you stay in agreement with God.

Here are some principles I follow when speaking affirmations:

I always speak my affirmations in the present tense as if what I believe already exists. I perceive my desired outcome as being real now.

My affirmations are always in the positive, not the negative.

I try to keep the affirmations short so I can focus my faith with strong conviction and clear thought.

When I speak my affirmations, I speak with force and confidence—releasing my faith through my words.

I use faith to fight fear, and I use my affirmations the same way. If I am feeling fearful or doubtful, I repeat the affirmations—alone, aloud, and with confident force. I always speak them at least one time every day.

Adjust them to fit your personal situation, but be sure to keep them in agreement with God's Word. Here are examples of affirmations I used when I had cancer:

I am a child of God and His promises are true for me.

God loves me and His plans are to give me a future and a hope.

God's Word is true and He is accomplishing His will in my life.

I am healed because of what Jesus did for me.

I give God full authority over my life—body, soul, and spirit.

I am healed according to God's Word.

I am vibrantly healthy.

Every cell in my body is functioning the way God designed it to function.

I am working in agreement with God's design for my body.

I am grateful to be alive and well, with a blessed future.

I recognize and accept the excellence of my healing plan.

With God's help, I am understanding the truth more every day.

Cancer has no authority to remain in my body.

My body is a gift from God—designed to heal itself.

I am helping my body heal every day by feeding it food created by God.

I repent for my actions that have damaged my body, and now I'm working with God to bring back healing and life.

I enjoy eating healthy foods . . . and I enjoy how healthy foods make me feel.

I eat to live healthy.

I am a faithful steward of the body God has given me.

I love to exercise and strengthen my body.

I live every day in gratitude and forgiveness.

I live a balanced life and enjoy every day.

My faith is strong because I believe God's Word is true.

I choose to spend one hour every day alone with God and His Word.

With God's help, nothing is too hard for me.

Endnotes

1. Isaiah 53:5

2. Dale's story is told in the bestselling book *Flight To Heaven* by Capt. Dale Black (Bethany House Publications, 2010)

3. Acts 10:34

4. Hebrews 13:8

5. Romans 10:17

6. Romans 6:23

7. Romans 5:8

8. 1 John 1:7

9. John 1:12

10. 1 Corinthians 10:13 AMP: "For no temptation (no trial regarded as enticing to sin), [no matter how it comes or where it leads] has overtaken you and laid hold on you that is not common to man [that is, no temptation or trial has come to you that is beyond human resistance and that is not adjusted and adapted and belonging to human experience, and such as man can bear]. But God is faithful [to His Word and to His compassionate nature], and He [can be trusted] not to let you be tempted and tried and assayed beyond your ability and strength of resistance and power to endure, but with the temptation He will [always] also provide the way out (the means of escape to a landing place), that you may be capable and strong and powerful to bear up under it patiently."

11. "Cancer Facts and Figures 2013," *The American Cancer Society, Inc.: http:// www.cancer.org/research/cancerfactsstatistics/cancerfactsfigures2013/ index* (July 14, 2013).

12. Ibid.

13. Robert Mendelsohn and Dr. Alan Levin, contributor, *Dissent in Medicine: Nine Doctors Speak Out* (Chicago: Contemporary Books, 1985), 82.

14. R. Webster Kehr, "Fourteen Questions and Answers about Cancer that Could Save Your Life," October 26, 2011, *Cancer Tutor: http://www. CancerTutor.com* (August 12, 2013).

15. Psalm 119:160

16. Dr. Barbara Starfield, MD, MPH, "Is US Health Really Best in the World?," *JAMA* (July 26, 2000).

17. Romans 10:17

18. James 4:8

19. Hosea 4:6

20. G. Edward Griffin, *World Without Cancer: The Story of Vitamin B17*, 2d ed. (Westlake Village, Calif.: American Media 2010).

21. Alan Scott Levin, M.D., *Dissent in Medicine: Nine Doctors Speak Out,* (Chicago: Contemporary Books, Inc., 1985), 82.

22. Mike Adams, "Massive Medical Fraud Exposed," July 9, 2004. *Natural News*: *www.naturalnews.com/001298.html* (September 5, 2013).

23. Ibid.

24. Marcia Angell, "The Truth About the Drug Companies," July 15, 2004. *The New York Review of Books: http://www.nybooks.com/articles/17244* (September 5, 2013).

25. R. Webster Kehr, "Introduction to Alternative Cancer Treatments," *The Cancer Tutor: http://www.cancertutor.com* (September 5, 2013).

26. Edward Griffin, *World Without Cancer: The Story of Vitamin B17,* 2d ed. (Westlake Village, Calif.: American Media, 2010), 22.

27. Ty Bollinger, *Cancer: Step Outside the Box,* 5th ed. (Houston, Tex.: Infinity 510 Squared Partners, 2010), 28.

28. Senate Bill 1828, Enacted December 23, 1971, *National Cancer Institute: http://legislative.cancer.gov/history/phsa/1971* (September 6, 2013).

29. Paul Raeburn, "National Cancer Program Called a Qualified Failure," (Los Angeles: May 29, 1985). *Associated Press: http://www.apnewsarchive. com/1985/National-Cancer-Program-Called-A-Qualified-Failure/id-4864109 300d970b97b8fa66f665642f1* (September 6, 2013).

30. "Linus Pauling Quotes," *Brainy Quote: http://www.brainyquote.com/ quotes/authors/1 /linus_pauling.html* (September 18, 2013).

31. 1 Peter 5:8

32. Rep. Louise Slaughter, "Slams FDA—Calls on agency to protect Americans health not industry profits," Washington D.C., February 2013. *Congresswoman Louise M. Slaughter Newsletter: http://louise.house.gov* (September 6, 2013).

33. Dr. Herbert Ley, *San Francisco Chronicle* (January 2, 1970)

34. Dr. Robert W. Christensen, *FDA, You Were Wrong! Stopping Innovation Stops America!* (Mustang, Okla.: Tate, 2012), 19.

35. Luke 15:4

36. Hebrews 11:1

37. Proverbs 23:7

Acknowledgments

Almost nothing in life is done strictly by oneself. All that we are and do is an accumulation of our faith, our family, our friends, and all who have touched our lives. It has taken two years to write this book; therefore, there are many people to thank. First, there are simply not enough words to thank God for His continued presence and faithful assistance throughout this process.

I also wish to thank my husband, Dale, for his love, his intensity of purpose, and his dedication to the truth. Without his involvement, this would have been a lesser book by far. We journeyed through cancer together . . . and together we revisited it.

Deep appreciation goes to a special friend and sister in Christ, Marianne Oelund. She believed in this book, followed her heart, and was used of God as an instrument to bring this project to timely completion.

There are many talented people to whom I would like to express my sincerest appreciation. Thank you to Karen Burkett, editor extraordinaire, who with the patience of a saint handled everything we gave her with grace and expertise. Great appreciation goes to her team of talent: Shannon Herring and Terri Hall, who faithfully put their ability and effort into helping make this book all it could be. A sincere thank you to Jerry Payne, whose remarkable editing skill and perceptive input added greatly to this book. Special thanks are extended to our daughter, Kara, who relived the story with us and contributed many valuable insights from her personal memories and discerning mind.

In conclusion, I wish to thank our dear mother, Joyce Black; our wonderful friends Scott and Lorraine Rogers; and our precious friend Dana McCue for surrounding us with encouragement throughout this process and believing in the message this book contains.

If the book *Life, Cancer and God*
has touched or stirred your heart and you would
like to share this message with others,
consider the following . . .

- Give this book as a gift. Touch someone else's life with a message of hope and inspiration.

- Share the impact—write a book review. Your favorite Internet places often supply a venue for your comments. You may also want to ask your favorite local radio show to do an interview or book review.

- If you have a personal website or blog, consider sharing something about the book and directing readers to www.LifeCancerAndGod.org.

- To order multiple copies of *Life, Cancer and God* at discounted prices, email your request to info@LifeCancerAndGod.org.

- Reach out and share with those in need by providing copies of the book to someone battling sickness or disease, your church library, or anywhere people may be encouraged and inspired by the story and its message.

- Encourage your church or organization to request the author as a speaker.

- Consider setting up a personal book study and inviting your friends and neighbors to meet together to read and discuss this book.

If you would like more up-to-date information and ideas on

how you can participate, check out the ***Life, Cancer and God*** page on our website: www.LifeCancerAndGod.org.

Visit us on Facebook at https://www.facebook.com/LifeCancerGod.

Feel free to connect by email: info@LifeCancerAndGod.org.

OTHER BOOKS by Capt. Dale Black

"Flight to Heaven—A Plane Crash . . . A Lone Survivor . . .
A Journey to Heaven—and Back"
A PILOT'S TRUE STORY by Capt. Dale Black
(Bethany House Publishers 2010)

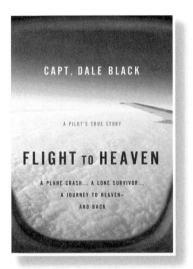

Flight to Heaven is a beautifully written and amazing account of life, death—and life again. In the early days of his flying career, Capt. Dale Black was a passenger in a horrific airplane crash that some have called the most ironic in aviation history. He was the only survivor. In the gruesome aftermath of the crash, Dale experienced a life-changing journey to heaven. This was not a vision or a dream, but a very real experience. Not only was Dale's life forever altered, but his story has also changed the lives of tens of thousands.

To those who have lost loved ones, this book is a source of deep comfort. It also gives readers renewed purpose and glorious hope for the future. This story is full of challenges and struggles that culminate in "overcoming faith" guaranteed to inspire.

To order an autographed copy of *Flight to Heaven,*
please visit http://www.daleblack.org/order-book.asp.

Reviews

Of all the books about heaven, this one's the best!
Tim Breuninger—San Diego, CA

As a publisher of four Canadian Best Sellers, a Search and Rescue Pilot, Photographer and Christian, I have found Flight to Heaven by Captain Dale Black one of the most inspiring books I have ever read! It is easy to read, factual and from the moment you start, you won't want to put it down. My wife and I ordered 15 copies for friends we love, just hours after finishing this amazing story.

Mike Biden—Retired SAR Pilot

Wow! Where do I even begin? The details of this book were so incredible that I felt as if I was on this journey as I read. This story has edified my faith that God is who He says He is and will do what He said He will do!! Aside from the Bible, this is by far the best book I have ever read!! It enveloped me from beginning to end. For anyone searching for the truth about this life or the afterlife, this book is for you.

Dana McCue—Memphis, TN

Next to the Bible, Flight to Heaven is the BEST BOOK I have ever read!

Pastor Shawn Machen—Sr. Pastor, World Victory Church

The whole world needs to read Flight to Heaven. I've had many authors on my radio show, but of all the NDE stories I've ever heard or read, Capt. Dale Black's is the best . . . by far!

Jeanne Jennay—Author and Radio Talk Show Host / Motivational Speaker

To say this is an inspiring book is an understatement. Flight to Heaven is an awesome read and has taught me a lot and given me peace and courage for a new chapter in my life. I'm purchasing more copies and giving it out everywhere.

Capt. Randy Hass—Airbus A320, US Airways

This "life after death" true story is both a page-turner and a faith-builder. The author does not commercialize his experience of heaven but tells it in a humble and reverent way while using breathtaking descriptions. I have recommended this book to my entire church.

Pastor Kenneth Cetton—Park Terrace Baptist Church

I could not put this book down and I cried through much of it. Flight to Heaven is the most moving and inspirational book I have ever read. And I do mean—EVER! After reading this book I am completely convinced Capt. Black's story is true and heaven is a real place.

Donna Benton—Syracuse, NY

I purchased this book as a gift for my dad, a retired airline captain, but soon discovered I couldn't put it down. Both of us are professional pilots and we easily rate it 5-Stars. The aviation aspects of the book are professional and technically accurate, yet the emphasis throughout is on a loving God. We think the book is a masterpiece and could be enjoyed by everyone, pilot or not.

Capt. E. Layton—Boeing 757, Major Airline Pilot

Dale's experience of the plane crash and trip to heaven has given him an incredible sense of looking at normal life through a spiritual lens and humble spirit. His commitment to Biblical truth and his ability to communicate from the heart as well as the head is admirable. Read this book and be prepared to be blessed in remarkable ways.

Pastor William Knopp, D. Min.—First Baptist Church of Corvallis, OR

To order an autographed copy of **Flight to Heaven**, please visit http://www.daleblack.org/order-book.asp.

ABOUT THE AUTHORS

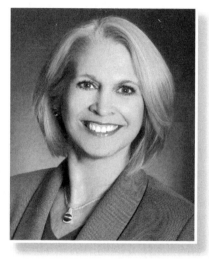

Paula Black is a wife and mother, businesswoman, author, Bible teacher, and seminar speaker. As the co-founder of Eagle International Ministries, she has helped lead teams of laypeople to many countries— preaching the gospel, offering medical aid, and distributing Bibles, gospel tracts, food, and clothing. She and her husband have helped build churches in several countries and established an orphanage in Guatemala. Paula speaks frequently at conferences and churches and has been interviewed on numerous TV and radio programs. Her unique ability to touch hearts has changed many lives.

Seventeen years after Paula reversed advanced-stage cancer naturally—without chemotherapy, without radiation, and without drugs—she shares her ONE-OF-A-KIND approach to health and healing of the *whole* person—BODY-SOUL-SPIRIT.

Paula grew up in Idaho and loves camping, fishing, and hiking, as well as golfing. Paula and Dale were college sweethearts and have been married since 1972. They have two grown children, attend Calvary Chapel, and live in Southern California.

Paula can be contacted at paula@LifeCancerAndGod.org or by visiting www.LifeCancerAndGod.org.

Capt. Dale Black is a husband and father, best-selling author, cancer researcher, Bible teacher, ordained minister, and former pastor. Dale has a BA degree from Point Loma Nazarene University, an MA in Theology, and a PhD in Business. He is a retired airline pilot instructor, jet captain, and aviation accident prevention counselor. Dale was the only 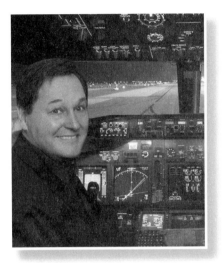 survivor of a horrific airplane crash. With massive life-threatening injuries, he used many of the principles described in this book to recover.

After losing dozens of friends and family members to cancer and having his wife diagnosed with advanced-stage cancer, Dale turned his research skills and his knowledge of God and the Bible toward understanding this horrible disease.

Dale leads the *Life, Healing and God* Workshops, where he and Paula teach their unique BODY-SOUL-SPIRIT approach to OVERCOMING sickness and disease, including cancer.

Dale can be contacted at <u>captdale@daleblack.org</u> or by visiting <u>www.daleblack.org</u>.

"If you hear the truth, will you believe it?"

— Paula Black